D0347301

The Nursing Process

THIS BOOK HAS BEEN ISSUED TO

GHN: gervis Pearson

AS A BENCH BOOK. DATE: Ward
April 1988

THE NURSING PROCESS

Charlotte R. Kratz, Editor

SRN,SCM,HVCert,DNT,RNT,BSc,PhD

Baillière Tindall
London Philadelphia Toronto
Mexico City Rio de Janeiro Sydney Tokyo Hong Kong

Baillière Tindall: 1 St Anne's Road
Eastbourne, East Sussex BN21 3UN, England

West Washington Square
Philadelphia, PA 19105, USA

1 Goldthorne Avenue
Toronto, Ontario M8Z 5T9, Canada

Apartado 26370—Cedro 512
Mexico 4, D.F., Mexico

Rua Evaristo da Veiga, 55–20° andar
Rio de Janeiro—RJ, Brazil

ABP Australia Ltd, 44 Waterloo Road
North Ryde, NSW 2064, Australia

Ichibancho Central Building, 22-1 Ichibancho
Chiyoda-ku, Tokyo 102, Japan

10/FL, Inter-Continental Plaza, 94 Granville Road
Tsim Sha Tsui East, Kowloon, Hong Kong

© 1979 Baillière Tindall. All rights reserved. No part of this publication may be
reproduced, stored in a retrieval system or transmitted, in any form or by any
means, electronic, mechanical, photocopying or otherwise, without the prior
permission of Baillière Tindall, 1 St Anne's Road, Eastbourne, East Sussex
BN21 3UN, England

First published 1979
Reprinted 1980, 1982, 1984

Printed in Great Britain by Spottiswoode Ballantyne Ltd, Colchester and London

---

British Library Cataloguing in Publication Data

The nursing process.
1. Nursing
I. Kratz, Charlotte R
610.73   RT41

ISBN 0-7020-0755-2

Contributors

Ian Hargreaves, SRN, RNT, FETC, Nat. Dip. District Nursing, Dip. Advanced Nursing Studies, MSc

Senior Tutor, In-Service and Post-Basic Education, Trafford Area Health Authority

Jean Crow, SRN, RNT, Dip. Advanced Nursing Studies, MSc

Tutor, South Manchester Schools of Nursing, Manchester

Janet Duberley, SRN, RSCN, Dip. Advanced Nursing Studies, MSc (Nursing Option)

Lecturer in Nursing Studies, Department of Human Biology and Health, University of Surrey

Karen Luker, BNurs., SRN, HVCert., NDNCert.

Research Training Fellow, Scottish Home and Health Department, University of Edinburgh

Contents

Introduction

This book is written by a group of nurses who have a number of things in common – an enthusiasm for nursing in its widest sense, a commitment to the problem-solving approach to nursing (the nursing process), and academic links. These similarities were important when planning to write this book.

Our common academic background convinced us of the need to approach nursing in a more logical fashion than had previously been done. This was interesting because most of us had been trained in ordinary nurse training schools and all of us had worked in a variety of posts within the National Health Service, some for a number of years. We were, therefore, not a group of starry-eyed idealists but had our feet planted firmly on the ground. But our experience in everyday situations had not blinded us to the fact that what was going on in our hospitals and in our community nursing services was not always perfect, and we wanted to be involved in improving it. We felt that the nursing process with its systematic approach to assessing a patient's needs, identifying problems amenable to nursing intervention and planning to meet them, documenting the nursing care given, and evaluating its effectiveness was a good way of doing it.

The fact that this approach to nursing was rapidly gaining acceptance from examining bodies indicated to us that we were on the right lines. It was, however, evident that this eminently appropriate way of nursing was meeting a considerable amount of resistance because it had originated in the United States of America, and the literature talking about it had been written by Americans. Unfortunately, nursing terminology written by Americans is not always familiar to us when it crosses the Atlantic. More important, although the logical approach to problem-solving is universal, the problems to which American nurse authors address themselves are not always similar to British circumstances: a different health care delivery system; the preponderance of one- and two-bed units in hospital, and the different preparation of nurse learners meant that the nursing process literature cannot be transplanted to these shores without difficulty. A book using familiar terminology and circumstances and by British nurses was urgently needed.

Writing such a book presented us with some difficulties. Because we had all learned about the nursing process through American literature, we had to make a conscious effort not to use expressions with which we had become familiar over time but which would not be readily understood by the British nurse learners. We hope that we have succeeded.

Adapting the book to the British nursing scene was rather easier. The authors had probably had as much, if not more, experience in using the problem-solving approach to nursing than any other comparable group of nurses in the United Kingdom. Not only were we familiar with it on a theoretical level, but we had been using or attempting to use it, in practice, teaching and research, not only in an academic setting but in the everyday setting of nursing practice and education. We knew about the problems from first-hand experience. We therefore hope that we have produced not only a readable book but a practical book.

Talking about the practical aspects of the book, it was only when reading the individual contributions that we realised how often (though not always!) our examples had been drawn from the practical sphere of nursing, from the 'helping with, doing' domain. This was in contrast to our theoretical stance, where we had spelled out our commitment to nursing as a helping, teaching, guiding profession concerned with emotional and social problems affecting health as much as with clinical problems. This stance, which directs how nurses use the nursing process, was very important to us all, and was the reason for our collaboration in producing this book. We knew that we all thought along similar lines – we were 'on the same wavelength.' We also knew that using the problem-solving approach to nursing without spelling out a new philosophy of what we understood by the term *nursing* would not bring the results for which many people hoped. We knew that nurses needed new problems to which to direct themselves, and not only new methods of solving old problems. We took our own common philosophy so much for granted that sometimes we almost forgot to transmit it to our readers.

However, the fact that so many of our examples were based on physical care, albeit on patient derived rather than on medically derived problems, probably also says something about the present state of nursing. The British nursing profession, including the authors, is so much more familiar coping with physical than with emotional problems that examples of the latter did not come easily. This is a worrying discovery, for nursing in order to survive has got to learn to meet the problems presented by its customers, or go under. The new philosophy of nursing, to which we all subscribe, is designed to meet the problems experienced not only by the acutely ill but by the growing army of people with handicapping and degenerative conditions who will consume ever greater amounts of nursing care, if we are prepared to give it.

It is probably true to say that all of us learned a great deal from writing this book. In fact, some of us felt that by the time the manuscript was completed we were ready to start on the second edition. This is probably no bad thing, for sharing our present state of knowledge with our readers should help them to achieve a fairly simple transition from 'nursing as it is' to 'nursing as it is going to be'. At the same time it should bring home to them that nursing is not a static activity but one that is continually changing. It is important to see that it changes in directions which we ourselves determine in accordance with what *we* see as being of benefit to clients or patients and do not allow others to tell us what we ought to do. That is why it is so important that nurses should, by using the nursing process, themselves identify the problems which their patients present, and decide on how they themselves want to meet them.

The book itself is written for nurse learners, though we hope that it will be found useful by nurses who, while qualified, want to learn more about the nursing process. The first chapter spells out the theory underlying the use of the nursing process, and we hope that the word *theory* will not cause readers to skip it, for we consider it an important chapter. Subsequent chapters illustrate the assessment, planning, care giving and evaluation stages of nursing process. We have tried to make them as practical as possible, using actual nursing histories and nursing care plans to illustrate our discussions. On the other hand, we have not suggested the use of any particular form of documentation for we think that this should arise out of the needs of specific nursing areas. Designing nursing histories and nursing care plans can help us more than anything to come to grips with our particular understanding of what nursing is about, provided we do not use it as a substitute for action. We finish with a chapter on the use of nursing process in the community nursing module to show that it can be used anywhere, provided it is suitably modified.

We have kept references out of the actual text so as not to inhibit the flow of reading, but we give suggestions for further reading at the end of each chapter.

It remains only to say that we were left in no doubt that the nursing process was a circular concept, each stage intermeshing with every other. We sometimes had difficulty in deciding where exactly to explain a particular concept, as it was important in more than one stage. Equally, it was important to make sure that another author had mentioned a concept which would be essential for explaining what went on at a subsequent stage of the process. However, we finally agreed that nursing process was less of a circle than a spiral, for we hoped that we should not return to our starting point again, but arrive at a point slightly higher than that. We hope that our readers will join us in exploring new heights.

The Nursing Process

1. Theoretical Considerations

There are a number of ways of looking at nursing. The view of nursing held by an individual, an institution such as a hospital, a unit in the hospital, or by society as a whole will determine the approach to the delivery of nursing care to patients.

One widely held view of nursing is that it is a reacting profession carrying out its activities in response to doctors' orders and under their directions. Indeed, much of what nurses do is related to, and is in response to, doctors' instructions. These so-called delegated functions of nursing contribute to the over-all objective of medical care, that is, to cure the patient. However, we as nurses make a contribution to the care of the patient which can be quite independent of the doctor. This independent function is well illustrated in the care of the terminally ill patient, who by definition cannot be 'cured' by medical treatment. The doctor's contribution to the care of this patient is mainly concerned with the prescription of medicines to relieve pain and suffering. These medicines are administered by nurses, who often have to exercise professional judgement in deciding when the medicines should be given to be of maximum benefit to the patient. The patient's physical and emotional care is, however, the direct responsibility of the nurses. That is the care that consists of comfort and support to patients and their family to ease them through the period leading to death and afterwards is provided mainly by the nurses.

Historically, the function of the nurse and doctor has not always been so closely linked as now. Prior to the technical advances in medical care and the growth of the hospital as the setting in which patients are cured of disease, most of the nursing took place in the home and was carried out within the family by relatives and friends. The growth of medical knowledge and the institutional-isation of medical care brought with it the need for a highly trained professional nurse as a member of a team trained to treat patients and their diseases.

Attention was focussed on the contribution of doctors in treating disease because of the significance of many of the advances in medical knowledge which became an integral part of the doctor's skill. Far less attention was given to our role as nurses in providing for the needs of patients and our role in helping patients meet needs created by the advances in medical knowledge.

This view of nursing results in a situation where all nursing care that is given is dictated by the doctor, and we may find that we spend our time carrying out procedures that the medical profession considers to be chores that can be carried out by less well-trained persons than themselves. The result could be that professional nursing would be concerned with such matters as giving the patient intravenous drugs, setting up intravenous infusions and making diagnostic visits to save the doctors' time. The patients' needs, physical and psychological, would be of little concern compared to the carrying out of these delegated tasks.

Florence Nightingale is regarded as the founder of modern nursing and the nursing profession as we know it today. It may be from her insistence that her nurses in the Crimea should do nothing for the patient unless instructed to do so by the doctor that this relationship between nursing and medicine grew. At that stage in the development of the nursing profession and in the situation in which those nurses found themselves it was probably the appropriate action to take. However, in view of the developments in the training of nurses one must question whether the statement made by Miss Nightingale in her book *Notes on Nursing* 'let no woman suppose that obedience to the doctor is not absolutely essential' still holds true. Obedience to the doctor in delegated functions is of course still essential, for example, giving of medicines prescribed by the doctor, at the times, and in the doses stated by the doctor. Even then nurses have a certain freedom to disregard doctors' orders if they suspect them of being wrong.

Florence Nightingale also cautions the nurse 'not to let the physician make himself head nurse'. This seems to indicate that she saw nursing as being only partly concerned with carrying out doctors' orders. She also recognised that there was much in nursing that was the nurses' concern and was controlled by the nurse and not the doctor.

What is Nursing Process?

The nursing process is basically a problem-solving approach to nursing that involves interaction with the patient, making decisions and carrying out nursing actions based on an assessment of an individual patient's situation. It is followed by an evaluation of the effectiveness of our actions.

Nursing process consists of a number of intellectual steps or thinking activities leading to nursing intervention. Actions are based on an assessment of the individual patient and are focussed through goals which are defined as a result of these steps. Stating the goals makes explicit what the nursing care is to achieve in terms of changes in the patient's situation. The nursing actions to be taken to achieve these goals are decided upon, using our judgement and such knowledge as we possess of the consequences of the proposed nursing care. The effects of our nursing actions are continually evaluated and reevaluated. If our actions do not achieve the set patient goals then an alternative action is adopted, or another goal set. Nursing process sets the patient firmly at the centre of the action.

Nurses are not alone in using a problem-solving approach. Doctors and other professionals also use this approach. However, the types of patient problem which they identify are different from those which nurses might identify. Essentially doctors identify medical problems and the emphasis is on the diagnosis of disease and its treatment and cure. The nurse does not focus solely on disease but on the meaning of hospitalisation and disease processes on patients and their families.

The nursing process consists of a series of steps which are carried out by the nurse and to explain it we must set out the stages separately.

The First Step

Assessing the patient to determine his or her need for nursing care or to identify problems that can be alleviated by nursing care is the first step. Those problems may be physical or emotional or social, but each one will affect the patient as a whole being. They may be identified by the patient or the nurse. Not every patient will have problems. Some may have a few, and a few patients will have many. Identifying a problem does not necessarily mean that it can be solved, either by nurses or by anyone else.

The Second Step
Planning nursing care by setting goals that will enable us to meet the problems which we have identified or to alleviate them if we cannot solve them is the next step. This involves deciding *how* the patient is to be nursed and communicating this to all the members of the ward team in the form of a *written nursing care plan*.

The Third Step
Nursing intervention, or carrying out the nursing care that we have decided may meet the patient's problems or solve them if possible, is the third step. This involves therapeutic interaction between the nurse and the patient, perhaps by listening to the patient or teaching the patient, as well as requiring technical competence such as giving injections, taking readings of monitoring equipment and the like.

The Fourth Step
Evaluating the outcome of our nursing actions to see whether the nursing care that we have given is *effective* is the final step.

It may appear that we always start at step one, assessment, and work through to step four, evaluation. It must be stressed however, that in practice each step is carried out continually. When we are caring for patients we are continually observing the patient and noting new problems as they arise and then taking the appropriate nursing action. We continually assess whether the nursing care we are giving is effective. If it is not effective, then an alternative way of dealing with the problem is adopted. The following example illustrates how the process works in the ward situation:

> An elderly patient is admitted to the ward in a very weak state. He is hardly able to move and is obviously thin, undernourished and dehydrated. However, there are no signs of redness or skin breakdown over his pressure areas.

This constitutes a simple nursing assessment of the patient. It is not a comprehensive assessment as much more information would be required to plan the total care of this patient. However, it is possible from the information in the example to identify some of the patient's problems as a basis for planning his nursing care.

Even the most junior nurse will have deduced that this patient is going to have a problem related to the prevention of pressure sores. We, as the nurses caring for this patient, will therefore have to decide how we are going to prevent pressure sores from developing. We will therefore make the goals of our nursing care 'to keep the patient's skin free from pressure sores'. We know that this may be achieved providing the pressure areas are not subjected to prolonged pressure. We also know that relief of pressure could be achieved in a number of ways. One method would be to turn the patient at regular intervals thus preventing sustained pressure on any one part of his body.

The assessment also reveals that the patient is undernourished. This indicates to us that the tissues are likely to be depleted of protein and therefore more susceptible to the effect of pressure. Replacement of tissue protein would help in the achievement of our goal to prevent pressure sores from developing.

Based on the preceding knowledge, we will decide on a plan of action. It may be that we decide to turn the patient on alternate sides every four hours and to give him protein-enriched fluids every two hours along with a high protein diet at meal times. This decision would be written down on the patient's plan of care so that all the nurses on the ward at any time of day or night would know exactly what they have to do to care for the patient effectively.

Each time the patient is turned we would observe the state of the skin over the patient's pressure areas. That is we would evaluate if the nursing care we are giving – four hourly turning and protein replacement – is achieving the objective we have set, preventing the breakdown of the pressure areas. If the pressure areas remain free from redness or signs of tissue damage then the nursing care is being effective.

However, if our evaluation indicates that despite four hourly turning the pressure areas are becoming red, that is, the goal of preventing pressure area breakdown is not being met, a reappraisal of the nursing actions is made and an alternative way of dealing with the problem is instituted. We may decide to alter the care plan to instruct the nurses to turn the patient every two hours, nurse him on a ripple bed and apply sheepskins to his elbows and heels. The effects of these actions are then evaluated.

The example illustrates how the nursing process ensures an ongoing and yet ever changing delivery of nursing care and how it enables our nursing care to be closely matched to the needs of the individual patient.

Some may feel that this description of the nursing process is exactly what all good nurses have been doing all the time. It is true to say that many nurses have used the steps of the nursing process when actually practising the art of nursing, but this has been done intuitively and not deliberately. As a result each nurse has had to make his or her own assessment of the patient and decide how to act in each interaction with the patient. Learners who were instructed by the ward sisters to carry out the nursing care were not able to see on what information the ward sister had based her decision to nurse a patient in a particular way or why she chose to alter the nursing care of the patient.

The use of the nursing process – which involves a systematic and deliberate assessment of the patient which is recorded for all the nursing staff to see and is updated as new information is obtained; the deliberate setting of goals to be achieved and a written plan of how they are to be achieved; and, finally, an evaluation of the effectiveness of all of the nursing care – makes it possible to show how decisions are made. This means that nurses are no longer carrying out sister's instructions with no understanding of how or why this relates to the particular patient for whom they are caring.

Although the stages in the process are set out in a particular sequence it must be stressed again that each stage may be returned to many times during the patient's care. In certain situations it may be inappropriate to begin the patient's care by sitting down and collecting information as part of a comprehensive assessment of the patient's physical and psychological state. If the patient has been admitted in a collapsed state and in severe pain as a result of an acute myocardial infarction, the obvious need is for a rapid assessment of the patient's problems in relation to maintaining circulatory efficiency. The immediate goal of the nursing care would be to maintain circulatory efficiency and relieve pain. At a later stage, once the immediate threat to life has passed and the patient is in the intensive care unit, a more detailed assessment of the patient would be carried out. This might uncover emotional factors that were causing the patient to be anxious, thus increasing stress and interfering with recovery. Appropriate goals aimed at removing the stress-causing factors would be set and the appropriate nursing actions taken. Their effect in relieving the stress would be evaluated by noting changes in the patient's condition. All the steps in the nursing process have been taken in this situation but at different times and to a greater or lesser degree in relation to each problem.

Because the nursing process involves the assessment of each individual patient by the nurse, problems can be recognised and thought through in a systematic manner. The nursing care is then planned to alleviate those problems, or better still, having foreseen difficulties, to prevent their occurrence. Once the nursing history has been taken the next step is to identify and define the problems.

Many problems can be identified by looking at the patient's general condition and may be obvious. If a patient is unconscious he or she will have a problem of maintaining a clear airway. The medical diagnosis will also help to identify problems needing planned nursing intervention, for example, a diagnosis of diabetes mellitus will indicate that the patient has a problem of metabolising carbohydrates. However, many problems will only be discovered by studying the patient's answers to the questions asked during the assessment or from things the patient may say to us while we are caring for and talking to him. He may perhaps mention that his wife is having problems in paying the mortgage while he is in hospital. Whether nurses consider this to be a problem which should concern them has yet to be decided.

The patient may present many problems or potential problems at any one time. The nurse will have to decide which problems have to be dealt with first and which can be safely dealt with at a later date. Not all patients will present problems in all areas that have been assessed and care must be taken to make sure that we do not infer problems that do not exist.

Having decided in which order to deal with the problems the nurse comes to the next stage, deciding what the nursing care is to achieve, the nursing goals. Using our knowledge of physiology, bacteriology, psychology, sociology and other sciences and our nursing skills, we shall have to answer the question of how we shall meet these goals. Having decided on a course of action we must go on to ask ourselves what the possible outcome of these actions would be. The answer to the second question is crucial. If the possible outcome is not going to meet the goals then an alternative action must be chosen.

Problems may be alleviated and the goals for care met in several ways. The problem of preventing pressure sores is solved by relieving pressure. This can be achieved in many ways; turning the patient, using a ripple mattress or patient support surface that spreads the body weight such as a water bed. The choice of the appropriate nursing action will vary according to each patient's needs. A patient with a fracture dislocation of the spine is especially prone to pressure sore development yet it would be inappropriate to nurse the patient on a water bed as the condition requires that he or she be nursed on a firm surface.

One specific nurse cannot possibly have all the knowledge to cope with all the problems that may arise. The solution to some problems may have to be sought from other nurses with different or greater experience, from nursing textbooks or from research studies on nursing care. The individual nurse's knowledge determines the degree to which he or she can identify patient problems, suggest solutions and carry out the nursing care to achieve the solution.

Once we have settled what the solution should be our decisions constitute the nursing orders which are written as the nursing care plan. This written care plan ensures that the nursing care of all patients is written down for everyone to see so that all who are caring for the patient are aware of the patient's problems and how they are being dealt with. The written care plan ensures also continuity of care throughout the patient's stay in hospital and provides an opportunity to plan in advance for any problems that may arise when the patient returns home. The care plan is updated as new problems arise or old ones are solved. It is an up-to-date plan of the patient's nursing care which changes as the patient's condition changes. However, we should realise that although we attempt to deal with patient problems and anticipate patient needs, the patient may be the best interpreter of what he or she needs and wants. It is therefore essential that we listen to what the patient is saying and take notice of it. It is important that we are able to distinguish between our own goals, values and standards and those that the patient is pursuing.

The nursing process is not in itself difficult to follow. The situations and problems that are identified may be complex and the over-all nursing care plan for some patients may be extensive, involving difficult and intensive nursing care. However, the basic steps in the nursing process can be carried out in any situation to enable the nursing care to be individualised.

Nursing is the outward and visible activities that the nurse does with, for, or on behalf of the patient. These actions are, however, based on a series of thought processes, such as assessing, identifying problems, setting priorities and choosing appropriate nursing care, which are not directly visible. These two together, the thought processes and the nursing actions, are called the nursing process.

The Nature of Nursing

Having given some thought to the steps which make up the nursing process, we must now return to our consideration of what we really understand by *nursing*. This is necessary because we state several times that nurses meet nursing problems. Fundamentally the steps of the nursing process are no different from the steps followed by anybody who wants to solve a problem. A man becomes aware of something that bothers him; he analyses it carefully, thinks of the best way to deal with it and then deals with it. In everyday life he will probably not stop to evaluate it consciously unless he has failed to deal with it, when he may ask himself what went wrong. But nurses would not necessarily consider themselves universal problem-solvers.

Problems are caused by unmet needs. Maslow identified man's basic needs, ordering them in a hierarchy. He started with those that were necessary for survival and finished with those connected with self-actualisation. In between came those related to safety, love and social esteem. He considered that you could not meet a higher need until the more basic needs were met. Many people never get beyond meeting those needs necessary for survival and safety, and though they may crave love and social esteem may never even give thought to the need for self-actualisation. In such an example we might say that the unmet needs for love and social esteem were causing such persons problems. On the other hand, the unmet need for self-actualisation was not causing a problem because the individual was not even aware of the need.

Problems, then, arise when we are unable to meet a need. Nursing problems arise when people are unable to meet certain health related needs. Virginia Henderson expresses this well when she writes:

> The unique function of the nurse is to assist the individual, sick or well, in the performance of those activities contributing to health or its recovery (or to peaceful death) that he would perform unaided had he the necessary strength, will or knowledge. And to do this in such a way as to help him gain independence as rapidly as possible.

It is important to realise that Miss Henderson here talks about activities which some people would consider 'non-nursing duties' and moreover says that these activities are *uniquely* nursing and therefore very important.

The nurse is concerned with helping the individual with things which he cannot do for himself and which are preventing him from carrying out his normal activities. The patient may be helped by the nurse actually providing those things for the patient. For example if the patient is unable to wash himself because, due to his illness, he has not got the necessary strength then we would wash the patient. However, the ultimate objective of helping the patient is to enable him to return to carrying out these normal activities himself as soon as he is able to do so. The example of the patient who has suffered a stroke illustrates the nurse's role in his care if Henderson's definition is accepted. He may be unable to wash himself, or feed himself due to paralysis of his arm. In the early stages of his illness we would wash and feed him. But if we hold the view of nursing expounded by Henderson, then we shall be concerned to see that the patient, as his condition improves, attempts to do these for himself. It would require us to consider how we can help him to learn to adapt to and cope with his changed circumstances, that is, only having the use of one arm. This would include providing equipment, or positioning equipment such as his bedside locker to enable him to reach his food or washbowl with his unaffected arm across his affected side. More than this, we would be concerned to see that he has the necessary time to carry out these activities for himself and that he receives support and encouragement whilst he learns how to cope in his new circumstances.

The nurse taking this view of nursing can be contrasted with one who considers that nursing is little more than meeting the physical needs of the patient and carrying out the doctor's instructions. She would approach the same patient quite differently. For example she would ensure that the patient received his medicines, she or an auxillary nurse would wash and feed him. However, the patient would never learn how to do these things for himself or be encouraged to try to do so, that is, he would never acquire the necessary strength, will or knowledge to carry out his normal activities again.

A view of nursing similar to that of Henderson is held by Orem who focusses attention on the role of the nurse in assisting the patient in those activities which enable him to care for himself.

These self-care activities are those that every individual normally carries out as part of his or her daily living and are related to meeting the basic needs for survival and functioning as a normal person in society. Inability to perform activities related to self-care arise as a result of injury or disease.

Both descriptions of nursing outlined suggest that nursing is primarily concerned with assistance to persons who are unable to help themselves in all or in specific areas of self-care. The assistance provided is in the form of doing something for or with another person to accomplish something that the individual would do for himself under normal circumstances. The nurse's ultimate objective would be to help the patient resume responsibility for the activity himself, when he has acquired the necessary strength will or knowledge. These two descriptions of nursing are useful in focussing on nursing actions, but are in themselves still insufficient to explain fully what is involved in nursing.

The Nature of Man

The practice of nursing will also be influenced by our assumptions about our patients, which in turn will depend on our view of the nature of man. Martha Rogers talks about these.

Assumptions about Patients and Environment that Influence Nursing Care

Individuals act as a unified whole

As we go about our normal activities, what we think, feel, experience, and do are all interrelated.

Consider, for example, how you have approached reading this book. You may have been instructed to read it by your tutor or read it out of interest because it was recommended by a friend. However, how you read it will be influenced by certain emotions that you alone experience and which are unique to yourself.

If you are sitting in a library that is cold, your efficiency in reading will be reduced. Because you as an individual act as a whole, feeling cold will interfere with the activity of reading and your ability to concentrate. Similarly if you had a piece of bad news earlier in the day your thoughts may be preoccupied with this and as a result your ability to read and concentrate on this book will be impaired. The same principle is illustrated by the patient who is extremely anxious about a particular procedure about to be performed on him. He may react in a manner that is totally out of character for him. He may become extremely angry and react by showing aggression towards a member of the nursing staff, his behaviour being the result of his reaction to the threatening situation.

Nurses unaware of the assumption about the wholeness of man would interpret this behaviour simply as hostility and dislike for that particular member of staff. However, nurses aware of the fact that man reacts as a whole, would see the situation as it really was – a total reaction of the individual to the threat and fear of an unknown and frightening procedure.

Similarly, a patient with a heart condition in which it is essential to rest, perhaps following an acute myocardial infarction, will be put to bed for complete bed rest. This reduces the demands on the heart by reducing the physical activity. However, because individuals act as a whole, complete rest will not be achieved if the patient is worried about something. He may be worried about himself, wondering if he is going to die, or about his family, or work. The patient will recover more quickly with complete rest only if the nursing care deals with the problem of his worry.

Nursing care *must be* concerned with the whole patient. No division can be made between the physical and emotional problems experienced by patients. Emotional problems will cause or may be caused by physical problems, just as physical problems will cause emotional problems.

Individuals are at all times influenced by the environment in which they find themselves

We learn to cope with particular environments, but changes in our environment can and do cause problems.

Remember how you felt when you began training as a nurse and entered the wards for the first time. The environment was new to you, and because you were new to nursing you did not know how to behave as a nurse in that environment. As a result you probably felt very frightened and anxious. Eventually as you learnt how to behave in and cope with this strange environment these feelings disappeared. The environment in which we find ourselves can also have a more direct effect on us and cause physical problems.

A person who has had a stroke and is left with a residual paralysis may have difficulty in returning to his normal environment, that is, his home, because he is unable to cope with such things as stairs, using the cooker or getting in and out of bed. On the other hand, the patient's environment may be contributing to his ability to cope normally with life. A person who has grown up with a permanent physical handicap will have organised his environment, his house, to compensate for his handicap. He will have the necessary equipment or modifications of his home to enable him to care for himself.

It is essential, therefore, that we direct our efforts not only to caring for patients, but that we do so with a full knowledge of how the patient's environment, both the hospital and his usual environment, affect him in terms of causing him problems or giving him strength. Our nursing care may at times be more appropriately directed at the patient's environment or his interaction with it. It may be necessary to assess the need for modifications in the patient's environment, or it may be concerned with teaching him how to alter his behaviour to cope with the environment in which he finds himself or to which he will be returning.

Environment can, however, also mean more than just the physical location in which we find ourselves. It is quite possible to talk about the social or economic environment in which the patient lives, and certainly about the psychological environment. If individuals are influenced not only by the physical environment in which they find themselves but also by the social and economic environment and particularly by the emotional one, then all these need to be taken into consideration when we are planning nursing care, for they may all influence the patient's health.

Behaviour is influenced by past experience
People's behaviour in a particular situation is influenced by their previous experiences, and their present experience will influence their future behaviour.

A patient who has been admitted to hospital previously and at that time experienced pain as a result of a particular procedure or treatment will be extremely frightened on a subsequent admission, as he will remember his previous experience and fear that a similar procedure will result in his experiencing that pain again.

Similarly, someone who suffers punishment at the hands of a person in authority may as a result of this experience resent anyone in authority and behave aggressively towards them. This effect of previous experience may become apparent when he is admitted to hospital where he could interpret the nursing staff as being in authority over him. His behaviour, influenced by his previous experience, may be to refuse to cooperate with the doctors and nurses and to show aggressive behaviour towards them. Without a knowledge of the patient's previous experience the staff are unable to control their interaction with the patient or give the necessary explanations to ensure that he realises that his previous experience would not be repeated in his present situation. The manner in which the patient is cared for on this occasion will also influence his future behaviour. If he is allowed to become dependent on the nurses during his stay in hospital then it is likely that this dependence will continue on his return home, and his relatives will bear the weight of his dependence, not the nurses.

However, the statement that man's behaviour is influenced by past experience has even wider implications. Unless we are dealing with a newborn infant, people have had various experiences which have helped to shape them into the sort of persons they are. It is unlikely that all children will behave alike, and certainly the older we get the more varied will have been our experiences before we entered hospital. Our reactions to hospital and the nursing care we require will depend on the sort of person we had become over time prior to admission. An old woman who has not been separated from her husband for the last fifty years will require different nursing care from one who has always lived on her own and liked it. Unless we take a patient's past experiences into account we are unlikely to provide appropriate nursing care. We should be aware of, and take account of the influence of the patient's past experience on his present situation and the effect of his present experience on his future.

Individuals have a normal daily routine and a number
of habits that are peculiar to them
All of us have a number of activities that we carry out each day and which we perform at more or less the same time each day. That is, we usually eat our meals at a certain time each day, bath or wash on arising or before retiring, have our bowels open each day or alternate days, and go to bed at more or less the same time in the evening.

Nurses must take into account the effect of disrupting this routine or attempting to interfere with the patient's usual habits (often acquired over a lifetime), on the recovery of the patient. For example, if a patient is noticed to wake every morning at 4 A.M. the night nurse might interpret this as inability of the patient to sleep. She would probably deal with this problem by asking the doctor to prescribe a sleeping tablet to be given to prevent the sleeplessness from recurring. However, had the night nurse been aware of the patient's normal habits and routine she would have known that the patient was a shift worker who habitually rose at 4 A.M. to start work at 5 A.M. The sleeping tablets would have been prescribed unnecessarily because the problem had been incorrectly identified, and the patient exposed to the risk associated with taking any drug without just reason.

Another illustration of how an awareness of the patient's normal habits and routine can increase the efficiency of nursing care is to be found in relation to elimination. Knowledge of how often the patient has a bowel action would help in planning nursing care to be effective if he should have problems in achieving a normal bowel action. If the patient usually has his bowels open on alternate days and immediately on rising, then the most effective time to help the patient who is constipated to have his bowel action would be on a day when he would do so normally and first thing in the morning.

Some people's habits may be seen by others to be idiosyncratic. For example, they may like jam with peanut butter or salt with porridge. Or on a more serious level, they may feel impelled to have a period of silence at night to read their bible, or to get out of bed and bow towards the East at regular intervals throughout the day. Others may never have gone to sleep in a single bed. While we may not always be able to ensure that patients may continue their habitual existence, knowing the alterations which being in hospital is imposing on them will help us to understand them better as people.

In planning nursing care for a particular patient a knowledge of his habits and usual routines will affect the type of nursing care we give and should help to make it more effective. If we disrupt a patient's routine we should at least be aware of doing so and not do it unnecessarily.

The interaction between two individuals influences
the behaviour of each
The way in which we interact with individual patients will influence the effectiveness of the nursing care in terms of their reaction to care and behaviour in response to that particular nurse. As nurses we should not only be concerned with the physical and emotional needs of the patient but should also relate to the patient as a person. We need to get 'under the skin' of the patient to see things as the patient sees them so that we have insight into the meaning of a situation for that patient as a person. Only

then are we able to help the patient effectively by planning our interaction with him or her. This ensures that what we say and what we do is done in such a way that patients learn that we understand them as individuals, who have particular and peculiar feelings and problems with which we may be able to help them because we understand what they are experiencing in relation to the problems or situation.

Thus far we have said that nursing is specifically concerned with health-related activities which patients would do for themselves were it not for some impediment in their situation. The way in which we would help patients with these activities would be influenced by our underlying assumptions about the nature of man. However, nursing is a complex activity, influenced not only by the preceding assumptions but also by being a helping relationship in which the nurse as helper relates to the patient to be helped as a person. We seek to help individual patients as people, not just to solve their problems related to their nursing needs.

We attempt to apply our knowledge objectively to the problems of the patient. Yet while remaining objective we still relate to the patient as a person as well as as a nurse. This implies that patients are involved in decisions about their nursing care. They are shown that they still have some control over what happens to them and the nurse respects their viewpoint. For this to be achieved they must be consulted and given the opportunity to agree or disagree with the proposed course of action. Throughout the patient's stay in hospital, the purpose of nursing care is to enable patients to deal with the problem themselves as soon as is practical, so as to become independent again as soon as possible.

The nurse may help the patient by:

a. acting on behalf of or doing something for the patient

b. guiding the patient in making a choice or decision about a particular course of action

c. supporting the patient by giving encouragement or motivating the patient to achieve something in order to reach independence

d. providing the environment that enables the patient to achieve certain goals and to become capable of carrying out things for himself or herself

e. teaching patients to do things that they had previously been unable to do or, which as a result of their illness they will need

to do to return to a normal way of life in their own environment
The care of most patients will require us to help the patient
by all or a combination of some of the methods listed.

The acceptance of the assumptions about man and his environment and an understanding of the helping relationship indicate
that nursing is much more than caring for a patient with a medical
diagnosis, giving treatments and medicines. The practical skills
which every nurse must develop are an essential part of nursing,
but they represent only the visible aspects. Underlying these visible
nursing activities are a series of intellectual processes based on
our assumptions about the nature of man and his environment,
and about the fact that nursing is a helping and enabling process.

If we think about a patient mainly as a person suffering from
some disease, then our questions to that patient will be mainly
about the disease, and our nursing actions will be directed only
towards curing that disease, usually by specific treatments or medicines. It is only when we spell out what we mean by nursing
in the way that we have attempted here that we realise that focussing
on the patient as a possessor of illness is not sufficient. Equally,
if we think of nursing only as doing technical procedures, we
shall not include nursing interventions in our nursing care plans
which may involve teaching, guiding or supporting the patient.
In other words, the content of a nursing history will depend on
our understanding of the nature of nursing for we might well
omit many questions unless we spell this out clearly.

The contents of a nursing care plan will depend equally on
our understanding of the nature of nursing, for even if we have
asked a great many questions, we may still not think that dealing
with the problems which we have identified is 'nursing'. Using
the nursing process in isolation will help us at least to begin
at the beginning and end at the end, something which nurses
have not always done. But it will not on its own improve the
quality and scope of nursing care.

The background knowledge we bring to bear on the patient's
situation as we understand it from a nursing assessment, enables
us to discover what each problem the patient experiences, or is
likely to experience, means to him or her. This type of understanding puts us in the best possible situation to help patients and
carry out their nursing care with a full understanding of their

needs and reactions to their present condition. Understanding patients helps the patients to trust the nurses who care for them. This trust, knowing what to expect from us and knowing what we expect of them allows the patients to participate in their own care. It prevents the situation where the patient fails to cooperate with the nurses because he or she does not understand what we are attempting to achieve.

Some people may think that dealing with anything but the immediate presenting problem in the way we have always done is unrealistic or Utopian, but there is enough evidence to show that unless we view nursing in the wider and more comprehensive way we have outlined here, the patient's return to optimum functioning may well be delayed. It is for this reason that this book will consider the use of the problem-solving approach to nursing – the nursing process – in this wider sense. Too many patient problems would remain undiscovered, and too many nursing actions remain undone, without it.

References and Suggested Further Reading

Davis, B. D. (1978) 'Why do we need the Nursing Process? For professional reasons.' Paper given at S.H.H.D. Nursing Research Advisory Group and reprinted in *Nursing Times*, Vol. 74, No. 48, pp. 1987–88.

Henderson, V. (1966) *The Nature of Nursing*. London: Collier-Macmillan Ltd.

Maslow, A. H. (1954) *Motivation and Personality*. New York: Harper & Row.

Orem, D. E. (1971) *Nursing: Concepts of Practice*. New York: McGraw-Hill Book Co.

Rediscovering the patient. A series of articles on the implementation of the Nursing Process in two centres in England. *Nursing Times Supplement*. 30 November 1978.

Rogers, M. E. (1970) *An Introduction to the Theoretical Basis of Nursing*. Philadelphia: F. A. Davis.

2. Assessment

Assessment is the first stage of the nursing process. The aim of this stage is to collect information about a person who is ill and then, by inspecting that information, to identify – and later to validate – the patient's problems.

Each stage of the nursing process is of equal importance to its over-all effectiveness of improving patient care. If we try to skimp on one stage it will be reflected in the quality of the next. However, this point is stressed particularly in the introduction to this chapter, as assessment forms the basis for the remainder of the nursing process. If insufficient time or trouble is taken over the assessment, fewer patient problems will be identified. This means that the second stage, that of constructing a care plan to assist the patient with his or her identified problems, will not be as comprehensive as it might have been. A nursing care plan, and nursing care generally, can only be as good as the information on which it is based.

Collection of Information

Part of the aim of the first stage of the nursing process was said to be to collect information about a person who is ill. Information about a person who is ill will include aspects of him as an individual, as a patient, as a member of a family, and as a member of a community. Such information is usually collected by means of a nursing history.

What is a Nursing History?

Nurses at present have no written guidelines on what information to collect from new patients, and this therefore results in great variations in the kind of information that is collected. The time given to collecting information from new patients also fluctuates in accordance with how busy nurses are. In contrast doctors, irrespective of how busy they may be, always find time to record a new patient's medical 'history. Nursing process requires that nurses place equal importance on the collection of nursing information as do doctors on collecting medical information.

When doctors take a medical history from a patient, they usually use a form that is divided into sections to remind them to enquire about and examine all the systems of the body, as well as to collect other relevant information, and with space to record their findings. Taking a nursing history also entails deliberate and systematic collection of information on predetermined topics, and recording this information early in the patient's stay in hospital. Such information will enable us to construct a personalised nursing care plan for the patient which will influence his care in hospital and allow more successful preparation to be made for his return back home.

If we are in any doubt about whether the system presently used by nurses enables us to prescribe personalised nursing care, we need only to read the information recorded on a nursing Kardex for a number of patients admitted with similar medical conditions. While, for example, ten patients admitted for breast biopsy will all require similar preoperative and postoperative treatment, each will also have a unique personality, individual fears and anxieties, all of which should influence nursing care. In other words, while they will all require an underarm shave and a premedication, the meaning of breast biopsy for a young unmarried girl, for a middle-aged woman and for someone nearing retirement may be quite different.

A nursing history focusses on the effect of the illness and of hospitalisation on the patient and his family, in contrast to a medical history which focusses on the illness itself. There should therefore be little information collected by nurses *and* doctors. A medical history is recorded to assist the doctor in making a medical diagnosis, and to guide the doctor in deciding on the optimum treatment aimed at curing the patient of the disease, or at least improving the patient. A nursing history is recorded to assist the nurse to identify the patient's problems and strengths and weaknesses, so that appropriate nursing care can be prescribed. All this will help the patient to function as adequately and independently as possible in hospital and when he returns home.

On the other hand, although a nursing and a medical history record different information and for different reasons, they are complementary as both are ultimately concerned with a patient's health. To guide us in deciding on the content of a nursing history we have therefore to consider what information is already available from the medical record, and also to attempt to define the unique contribution the nurse makes in the health care team, so that this could then be used as the framework for constructing our nursing history.

The World Health Organization defines health as a 'state of complete physical, mental and social well-being, and not merely the absence of disease or infirmity'. These three components of health (or well-being) – physical, mental and social – should not be considered in isolation, for they interact at all times. For example, students will readily appreciate that physical tiredness from late nights or anxiety resulting from a broken personal relationship can easily affect their performance in an examination. A girl with anorexia nervosa may require psychiatric treatment, yet could die from starvation. A man with idiopathic epilepsy may have difficulty in finding suitable employment, not only because of his medical condition but because of the social stigma attached to it. A nursing history therefore needs to enquire into all three components of health. The unique contribution of the nurse to the health care team is defined as

> assisting the individual, sick or well, in the performance of those activities contributing to health or its recovery (or to peaceful death) that he would perform unaided if he had the necessary strength, will or knowledge and to do this in such a way as to help him gain independence as quickly as possible.

Assisting patients to gain maximum independence if cure is not possible, or helping them to have a peaceful death is in keeping with the changes in the pattern of much ill health nowadays. Today, the greatest health care needs are not met with life-saving drugs and techniques, but with improving the quality of life of those patients who may have incurable and degenerative conditions. When there is nothing more to do medically for a patient, nurses continue to be able to provide a great deal in the way of nursing care.

The words *strength*, *will* and *knowledge* in the definition cited correspond closely to the nurse's triple role of physical helper, emotional supporter and teacher. For example, adequate physical care is needed if an unconscious patient is to survive. A woman having had a frozen section of a lump in her breast followed by mastectomy may need tremendous emotional support to help her overcome her fears of reduced femininity and of knowing that she has a life-threatening disease. A patient who has been newly diagnosed as having diabetes may need to be taught how to inject his own insulin, perform urinalysis, calculate his daily calorie intake, and how to care for his health generally to help reduce the risk of possible complications.

Having looked at the components of health, and at the unique contribution of the nurse in the health care team, we can see that a nursing history should record information on the physical, mental and social aspects of a particular patient's well-being, or lack thereof, so that we can then identify ways of giving physical, emotional and informative support, until such time as the patient recovers from his illness, accepts and adapts to his remaining disability, or dies.

The Content of a Nursing History

A nursing history might assess some or all of the following areas:
Personal information
Information on the present illness
Experience of previous illnesses
Personal lifestyle
Social and interpersonal information
Medical, nursing and social care received prior to admission for present illness
Planned medical care for present illness
A systematic physical, mental and functional assessment

These areas give a basic structure to a nursing history. In addition it is useful to have space for recording any concerns or worries expressed by the patient during the taking of the nursing history, for observations made by the nurse while taking the history – which may either add to the information provided by the patient, or

Personal Information	Social and Interpersonal Information	Physical, Mental and Functional Assesment
Information on Present Illness	Medical, Nursing and Social Care	Observations
Experience of Previous Illness	Planned Medical Care for Present Illness	Summary of Immediate Problems
Personal Lifestyle	Additional Information	

Fig. 1. Outline of a nursing history.

throw doubt on some of it – and it is also useful to have space for a summary of the main points which have been discerned. A rough outline of a nursing history could resemble Figure 1.

Therapeutic concern and *not* idle curiosity should govern the collection of information from any patient. This means that we only collect information which will be positively useful, but does not imply that we should feel obliged to meet, let alone solve, every problem which we do identify. Knowing that insoluble problems exist may sometimes help the patient as well as ourselves.

Personal information

Much of the personal information, such as the patient's name, age, address, next of kin and the like, will already be available from the medical history. Nevertheless, they should also be recorded on a nursing history, not only because of the actual information which they contain but because of the opportunity they provide for a double check. Many nurses will be able to relate stories where on second asking the patient may admit to having given inaccurate information, for example, about age, and although age is a poor indicator of a person's health and ability, not admitting to one's age may uncover all sorts of underlying problems. Furthermore, it may help us to modify some of our expectations. Quite often, too, patients will give an address which may either not have been the address from which they were admitted or may not be the address to which they plan to return after discharge. Accurate personal information will also reduce the possibility of error, for example, sending someone else's notes or X-rays with the patient to the operating theatre, or increase a favourable opportunity such as celebrating a birthday! Information on the next of kin, or perhaps even the fact that the patient was too ill to provide the personal information and that it was provided by someone else, will be of particular importance to nurses, some of whom are usually available when relatives visit, require information or reassurance, or when we wish to make arrangements for future care.

Information on the present illness

Many nurses would argue that information on the present illness is also readily available from the patient's medical notes, and that asking patients about their illness will provide less accurate and reliable information. However, not only do patients like talking about their illness and therefore appreciate an opportunity provided for this purpose, but often the fact that they have inaccurate information or unrealistic expectations about the course of their illness or unnecessary fears are of immense importance for the subsequent course of the illness. Without this kind of information we are unlikely to fulfil adequately our roles as emotional supporters and givers of appropriate information, however skilful our physical care of the patient may be.

Experience of previous illnesses
Again it could be argued that information on previous illnesses is already available, but there are many instances where patients have forgotten to tell the doctor some detail of a previous illness episode and now worry whether it matters or not. Nurses want to know additional details other than diagnoses and treatments, they want to know whether the patient has any particularly pleasant or unpleasant memories of previous illnesses or admissions to hospital. For example, a patient may recall being in a side ward and being very lonely, or he may recollect feeling embarrassed by the doctor asking personal questions in a loud voice, or how he was prepared for surgery and then the operation being cancelled. Some remember investigations which they found particularly unpleasant, and they can sometimes be assured straight away that these are now carried out in a different manner.

Many patients also have happy memories, of how kind sister was about visiting, of the good food and the like. Knowledge of previous admissions equips us to utilise the positive and avoid or bear in mind negative memories. If a patient has not previously been in hospital, then the patient will need additional information about visiting, who is who, or perhaps on how to ask questions or even to complain.

Personal lifestyle
Information about a patient's activities of daily living should be collected, which include items such as sleep, personal hygiene (that is, how often a patient usually has a bath, or if he prefers a shower, or if he normally cleans his teeth after every meal

or not at all), bowel and bladder habits, how far the patient can and does walk. It is also useful to know who usually provides his meals, does the cleaning and shopping and the like for all these will affect the stage he will have to reach before he is ready for discharge. Such information is also useful as often patients will talk about what they could do, and do not differentiate between the immediate and the more distant past. Knowing what patients could do prior to their present illness enables us to try and minimise changes resulting from the present illness, and to show greater understanding towards patients whose lifestyle has been drastically changed by a sudden catastrophic illness such as a stroke. Assessment of this aspect of a patient's existence is of particular importance to nurses, for much nursing care is directed towards helping the patient in just these areas. These areas are the particular concern of nurses, and if they are neglected by us, they are unlikely to be attended to by anyone else.

Social and interpersonal information
Social and interpersonal information about the patient's family or friends, work, leisure and accommodation will need to be collected. Should the patient have come to hospital unaccompanied, the next of kin to be informed will have to be established. However, the size of the patient's family, where they live in relation to the patient, how often they see each other, their ages, occupations and often their state of health will all add to the total picture of the patient as a unique being. Some patients have no family, or indicate few concerns about them, but may be worried about not having locked up or not having made arrangements for feeding the budgerigar. They accept treatment more willingly if we can reassure them that arrangements are being made about dealing with these problems for them.

Knowing a patient's occupation will give some indication as to his economic situation and possibly also to his educational attainment, and may influence what and how the nurse will teach the patient aspects of his care. Wherever possible our teaching should take account of these points, for it is often inappropriate to give advice which will go counter to these, and there is much evidence to suggest that patients do not follow instructions which upset their usual way of existence. Furthermore, there may be some newly diagnosed condition which is not compatible with the patient's normal occupation, and drawing early attention to such a possibility and supporting the patient who may have to come to terms with such an upheaval in his life may be an important part of nursing care.

Patients' pastimes may again provide some indication of their socioeconomic and educational background and of their way of life generally. The patient who enjoys active outdoor pursuits will react differently to a period of enforced idleness indoors from one whose great wish has always been to have enough leisure to catch up on his reading. Those who enjoy watching TV and listening to pop music require different arrangements from those who like knitting and chatting or who just like to sit quietly doing nothing.

For the nurse in hospital one of the most important points on which to gather information is about the patient's accommodation – where he lives, the kind of amenities available both inside and outside, and the problems which he perceives such accommodation to pose in his existing situation or which he fears may become apparent as a result of his illness. Does he live in a flat or a house? Are there steps to climb, what are the cooking and heating facilities? Is it his own, does he pay rent or has he a mortgage? Availability of facilities such as buses and shops will indicate whether a person is housebound due to lack of mobility, of services or because of financial problems. Some information about neighbours, helpful or otherwise, could also prove useful.

While we would expect to have established the patient's religious affiliation when asking for other personal details, an inquiry of how important this is to him may not be out of place when investigating his social environment. Only in this way can we respect his taboos or organise the provision of extras such as special diets, visits by the hospital chaplain or appropriate religious leader, which make all the difference between routine and individualised nursing care.

Previous medical, nursing and social care
Knowing something about patients' relationship with their GP may indicate not only their normal state of health but whether they are people who frequently seek professional support or who prefer

to rely on their own resources. Often patients bring in their own medicines and then it is important to know what they are so that we can ensure that the appropriate drugs have been ordered by the houseman or more importantly so that we can act intelligently when dealing perhaps with a patient's constipation or with relieving pain in a patient who over many months has learnt to control it himself. Finding out about the drugs patients normally take may also provide us with an opportunity for checking their knowledge of their dose and action and providing remedial teaching if necessary.

Often patients, particularly those with long-term illnesses or who are elderly, may have been receiving nursing care and social services at home. If patients do not bring a nursing history and care plan with them on admission, information may have to be sought from the staff who have been looking after them at home, and contacting them before patients are discharged is vital. The same applies to social services, who often require notice some time in advance if they are to restore services which have been withdrawn on the patient's admission to hospital.

Planned medical care
An outline of the planned medical care is essential as many nursing actions are derived from medical treatment. For example a patient who has a fractured tibia may have a full leg plaster of paris applied as part of his medical treatment, and the nurse will be required to observe the limb for evidence of circulatory impairment. A patient whose diabetes is unstable may be ordered to have soluble insulin four hourly, to be adjusted in accordance with the amount of glycosuria and ketonuria present. It will be the nurse who decides the dose of insulin to be given based upon her accurate urinalysis and it will be the nurse who actually administers the insulin. A patient in congestive cardiac failure may be prescribed a diuretic for his generalised oedema and a digitalis drug for his atrial fibrillation as part of his medical treatment, but the nurse plays a vital role in maintaining the effectiveness of the drugs by recording an accurate fluid balance and by observing the relationship between a patient's pulse rate and apex beat.

The patient's usual activities of daily living may also be affected by the planned medical treatment, so this information is necessary before making a care plan for a patient. For example, orthopaedic patients requiring traction as part of their medical treatment will be confined to bed, and thus dependent on the nurse making provision for facilities for washing, eliminating, eating and the like. Patients who have recently had a myocardial infarction may be ordered complete physical and emotional rest as part of their medical treatment. They too are confined to bed and not only require provision for facilities to be made available as stated above but require the nurse to perform or assist them with their use.

Physical, mental and functional assessment
By using our special senses we may systematically assess patients' physical and psychological states and their ability to function normally. Observations made of each system would help to guide us in prescribing appropriate nursing care. Such observations are often made in a piecemeal fashion already. However, when using the nursing process, these observations are made systematically and consciously. Omitting an observation becomes a conscious act and not one based on oversight. Similarly using a list of adjectives describing a patient's mood is a way of consciously assessing and recording a person's state of mind, which should be taken into consideration when planning that patient's care.

A functional assessment differs from a straight physiological assessment in that it estimates whether an observed loss or abnormality hinders the patient in functioning normally. For example, a person may have only one leg, but manage to get about with ease on his artificial one. The functional assessment would therefore identify no problems of locomotion. Similarly a patient may be rather hard of hearing. Providing her with a hearing aid may be all that is required to allow her to function at an acceptable level. On the other hand, if she does not know how to regulate it or how to replace spent batteries or feels embarrassed to have to wear it and therefore keeps it in her locker, she will remain hearing impaired.

None of these assessments requires us to be able to manipulate elaborate pieces of machinery.

Additional information
The information collected under the various headings provides us with the kind of information which will enable us to see patients

as more than a diagnostic label requiring the administration of prescribed treatment. They will have become living, sentient beings who require information, help and support to enable them to come to terms with their particular illness related problems. For this reason, because every patient is also an individual, we can never fully predict the outcome of information collection. We shall therefore never be able to predict *all* the information to be collected, so it is useful for a nursing history to contain space for 'other' information – information which the patient may have volunteered in the course of the interview, or answers to supplementary questions which we may have added as we became alerted to a patient's special personal concerns. It may also be useful for indicating what patients considered their most urgent problems, which may be different from the ones we considered most urgent, but which will have to be met before the patient will be able to settle down to the business of getting better.

Observations made while taking the history
The observations we make while taking the history are different from the systematic observations about the patient's condition made as part of a nursing assessment. They may be concerned with the non-verbal aspects of communication – the patient who assures us that he is not worried in the slightest while sitting on the edge of a chair twisting his fingers; the patient who obviously did not wish to answer certain questions addressed to her or who seemed to be confused and inconsistent in her answers; or the patient who deliberately gave inaccurate information, for example that he never or 'hardly ever' smoked yet appeared to have heavily nicotine stained fingers. Further enquiry, possibly at a later date, might be necessary to sort out the discrepancy between verbal and non-verbal communication.

Summary of Main Points
By now a great deal of information may have been collected about a patient. While all this is essential for preparing adequate and comprehensive care plans, this latter activity may take some time, and in the meantime it is useful by means of a summary to identify those areas requiring immediate intervention. The summary is however not a short cut to avoid reading all available information.

Format of a Nursing History

If all the information about a patient which we have collected is not to be forgotten, and moreover is to be available to other nurses, who may be responsible for his care when we are off duty or otherwise not available, it is essential that it be written down. Also unless our original assessment has been committed to paper, it will be impossible to demonstrate the rationale for our care plans or to identify, when we reach the evaluative stage, why we may not have been successful in meeting our objectives.

Let us examine briefly three ways of recording a nursing history: self-recording by the patient; structured interview; and semistructured interview.

Self-recording by the patient

A useful way of getting routine information from patients and one which may save considerable nursing time is self-recording by the patient. It may be particularly useful in areas having a large number of routine admissions. The patient is given a questionnaire asking for the sort of information which he can easily give about his personal circumstances, as well as about his illness. It may be possible to send such a questionnaire to the patient prior to admission and ask him to bring it with him when he comes in. He may even like to fill it in with the help of his family or workmates.

However, there are certain disadvantages to making patients complete their own nursing history form. Firstly, it prevents any real interaction between patient and nurse on admission, and may thus seriously stunt the development of a beneficial nurse-patient relationship. Secondly, patients may write what they think we want to hear rather than 'the facts' whether they think these too creditable, or too discreditable. During an interview we are likely to pick up some clues indicating such incongruity, but unless we talk to the patient in addition to collecting his completed questionnaire, we shall miss these. While, therefore, a self-recorded patient history is better than no history at all, it should, whenever possible, be supplemented by at least a short interview.

The structured interview

In the structured interview nurses have decided the information they will require as a basis for planning nursing care. The history format therefore consists of a number of predetermined questions, usually in a set sequence, to which the nurse collects answers. This format has the advantage of speed and completeness. Writing is reduced to a minimum, and if a question is not answered it is due to a deliberate decision – either by the nurse not to ask it or by the patient not to reply. Unless, however, a section for additional information is added to such a format, it may again lack completeness as already indicated.

The semistructured interview
In a semistructured interview the history format may consist either of a frontispiece containing a list of areas to be explored with the patient during the interview or the areas may appear as discrete headings rather as shown in Figure 1. In either case, the nurse checks that she has covered all the areas indicated, but there is no indication whether information which has not been recorded has not been collected or whether there was no relevant information to record. It will be appreciated that using a semistructured approach will give the patient great freedom to explore the areas which he himself considers important. On the other hand, it is time-consuming for the nurse, and may, in addition, lack completeness.

In practice it may be best to aim for a combination of all three methods, allowing patients to complete their own questionnaires as far as possible, checking this information with them, and at the same time collecting additional predetermined data, and also allowing free expression of concerns in areas which the patient himself determines. Until nurses are very familiar with taking a nursing history, allowing a completely semistructured or unstructured approach will probably give least satisfactory results for omissions will be too great, and it would be simple to return to the present unsatisfactory Kardex system.

Some people may wonder why we have not spelled out in minute detail the content of a nursing history. The decision not to do so was deliberate. While we illustrate a number of formats which have actually been tested and used in a number of wards in chapter 3, we consider a nursing history to be both specific to a particular area and dynamic in that it should be easy to make at least minor adjustments to its content and layout. We hope that nurses will experiment with adapting outline formats to suit the specific needs of the patients in the area in which they work, rather than follow slavishly a specific example.

Timing a Nursing History

The assessment stage forms the foundation for the remaining stages of the nursing process. This means that personalised nursing care cannot be planned until information about a new patient has been collected. It would therefore seem logical that we need to record a nursing history at the earliest opportunity following the patient's admission. In the real world, however, there are frequently intervening factors that may make us modify the implementation of the ideal. These intervening factors may be patient-based or nurse-based.

Patient-based factors

The patient may be in no physical condition to participate in the interview. For example, he may need to have his airway maintained, fluids administered, bleeding controlled, shock treated, or pain controlled. On the other hand, he may simply need rest or food. Diagnostic tests and treatments may in some patients have priority. If the patient has already been interviewed, perhaps by a doctor or the police following an accident, the nurse may feel that her own interview could with advantage be delayed for a while. On the other hand, the fact that a doctor (or a medical student) arrives while the nurse is taking a nursing history does not necessarily mean that she should stop. Quite apart from the damage such an action might do to a developing nurse-patient relationship, she may well be collecting information of as much use to medical staff as to herself, and certainly of as much importance to the patient. Taking a nursing history may therefore be delayed until the patient can participate effectively and with no danger to himself.

Patients who are confused or aphasic or perhaps young children who are not accompanied by a member of their family or a friend may also need to have the nursing history interview postponed until relatives are available to give the necessary information.

Nurse-based factors

One factor which may delay taking a nursing history is the number of staff on duty. At times other patients may have such overriding needs that they must be attended to before a nursing history is recorded for a new patient. Emergency admissions can cause unexpected staffing shortages, and although a nursing history will be taken it must of necessity be short until the immediate crisis is over, as nurses have a duty to all the patients on a ward for whom they are responsible.

Inadequate staffing levels may however be used as an excuse for not recording nursing histories. If a nurse is not convinced of the importance of this procedure or is unskilled in recording a nursing history, it is not difficult to find other things to occupy her time. In no case, however, should taking a history be delayed for more than twenty-four hours.

If nursing histories are to be considered a legitimate part of every patient's nursing care, then time must be allocated to recording them. Without systematic collection of adequate information nursing care can become ritualistic and inappropriate to the needs of a particular patient.

So far little attention has been given to identifying the areas in a nursing history which are *critical* for the delivery of quality patient care. Perhaps when identifying the content of a nursing history for a specific area as previously suggested, thought might also be given to indicating information which *must* be collected immediately and that which can wait if necessary. We would like to add at this point that as with everything else, taking a nursing history becomes easier and quicker with practice.

Taking a Nursing History
In order to collect such comprehensive information about a person who is ill we need to utilise several different sources. The most lucrative source for collecting information about a patient as an individual is the person himself. Additionally, as the dictionary defines a patient as 'a person under medical treatment' information on the person as a patient would involve searching the hospital medical records as well as looking for any communication from the community health services. Talking to the patient's relatives would allow information about the person as a member of a family. Information on the patient as a member of a community can be collected by talking to visitors, such as friends, colleagues from work, or others interested in the patient.

Record-searching

Searching of records refers to any written information concerning a patient. The advantage of such records is that written information is stable and therefore available for reexamination.

We shall first need to know where the patient's notes can be located in a particular area, and how to recall notes from an earlier admission. The notes may contain information about the patient from the source of referral, for example, the outpatient department, another unit, hospital, or the community health services. They may also contain the patient's current medical history with a conclusion as to the suspected medical condition, planned medical treatment including tests to confirm the diagnosis, and a progress report about the patient's response to outpatient treatment.

Only when we are familiar with the organisation of medical notes can we become efficient at searching them for the information of particular use to ourselves to assist in compiling the nursing history. In future, retrieving records for patients who have been previously admitted should also provide us with information about their nursing care from previous nursing histories and care plans. However, no factual information should be transferred from existing records to new ones, as too often data concerning the patient such as his address may have changed.

Interviewing the patient

By recording a nursing history baseline information is collected about a patient. The richness of the information contained in a history depends to a large extent on our skills as interviewers. We shall therefore need to know how to prepare the physical environment for conducting an interview, and how actually to conduct the interview.

Preparing the environment   Points for consideration when preparing the physical environment for an interview may be the seating arrangement, reducing interruptions to a minimum, and providing privacy. Making sure that the patient is sitting comfortably, either facing us or else sitting parallel to the interviewer, is important. It is important that the patient should be able to feel that he can relax. If at all possible interviews should be conducted in a room free from interruptions, preferably where we can shut the door, and even hang up an 'engaged' sign, though we must bear in mind that some patients may feel intimidated by too much formality. Whenever possible, information about the patient should, however, not be collected by the bedside, where only the curtains provide a semblance of privacy, and where we know that it is only too easy to be overheard by the patient in the next bed. If taking a history with the patient in bed is unavoidable, this should also be kept in mind.

Anyone who has ever been a patient will appreciate how lying down gives us a feeling of powerlessness, similar to being in the dentist's chair. To help avoid this feeling, it is best to sit down by the bedside. This indicates to the patient that we are there to stay and listen, and are not preoccupied with other activities.

Interviewing skills Some nurses assume that a patient will feel uncomfortable at having to be interviewed, and at the nurse making notes during the interview. Nurses who have actually recorded a nursing history will know that they, too, can feel some discomfort.

A knowledge of certain aspects of non-verbal communication will help us when conducting an interview. For example, gestures in the form of intermittent head nods while the patient is speaking, indicate that the nurse is listening, and that the patient has permission to continue. Such a gesture can be used by us to encourage the patient to continue speaking, or it can be used to redirect the interview.

Eye contact, when used in crowded conditions, can often be embarrassing. Eye contact between ourselves and our patients, when not encroaching on their personal space, can be used to assure the patients that we are primarily interested in them, and therefore affects the type of information entrusted to us. This requires also that we need to be familiar with the nursing history format if we are to focus attention on the patient and not on filling out the form.

A technique which may reduce discomfort both of ourselves and of the patient is to sit facing the same way as the patient. That way the patient can see what the nurse is writing, which may give a sense of working together, and also reduce the sense of secrecy which often surrounds health records. Where arrangement for interview does not permit shared visibility of the record, then commenting aloud on what we are writing decreases the patient's feeling of exclusion. Another way of reducing the discomfort felt by both parties is by explaining the reason for writing. 'I'll make some notes of what you tell me so that I can refer to the important points later to help me decide on the nursing care you need'. Recording the information after we have left the patient can easily result in inaccuracy.

While conducting an interview we need to be aware that collection of information is a two-way process. We need to realise that just as we shall use our baseline information about the patient for subsequent planning of his nursing care, so too the patient will modify his expectations about the nursing staff on the information collected from us.

The ability to record information as it is collected is a skill that has to be learned. Once learned it can give the patient a sense of involvement and create a climate of trust.

Once a nursing history has been recorded we have to decide where to file it. One school of thought is that if the patient has seen what we have written, then there is no reason why the nursing history cannot be left by the patient's bed. Another approach is that the nursing and medical history should be filed together. This would make available a comprehensive account of the patient's health-related problems, which would be of use to all concerned with the care of him.

Whichever filing method is used, the problem of confidentiality of notes remains. However, this problem is not a product of the nursing process, as our present system already allows a patient's notes to be transported by theatre porters and others within the hospital. Confidentiality of notes must be assured regardless of who has collected the information which they contain, and it is unlikely that a nurse's notes are more potentially harmful than those of a doctor.

It is often thought that recording a nursing history is a time-consuming business. However, as the present system of collecting information is so haphazard, we are unable to quote how much time is involved in this process, so that it is difficult to make comparisons. It may be useful to allow a student to take a patient's nursing history, while a colleague compares the information she obtains with what has been recorded in the   twenty-four hours. Few nurses fail to be convinced of the value of the new system after that. And, most nurses are surprised when patients say that they actually enjoyed being interviewed.

Observations

A factor which will affect the richness of the baseline information contained in a nursing history is our observational skill. Observation, being a descriptive process, requires receiving cues through our sense organs. By utilising as many sense organs as possible in a given situation we can observe the information the patient is communicating to us not only verbally but also non-verbally. Enriching nurses' observational skills will require the development of the comprehensive use of all sense organs, knowledge of certain aspects of verbal and non-verbal communication and consideration of factors which may influence recording one's observations.

Most nurses think that they are observant by nature, or if not observant by nature that their training has made them so. However, it may be worthwhile to try and think back no further than the most recent lecture by a new lecturer which we attended, and try to remember not just its content, but details about the lecturer. What was her hair colour and style? What jewelry, if any, did she wear? Did she have a wedding or an engagement ring? Did she have any specific mannerisms, like saying 'er' a number of times? What did she bring into the classroom with her, was she lefthanded or righthanded? Did she appear happy or unhappy, and what cues indicated her state of mind?

Having discovered that we are not as observant as we thought, we may also realise that so far we have only used our eyes. Yet the use of touch, hearing and smell all contribute to compiling a picture of a particular individual, and in the case of a sick person may bring us vital information. Our nose should help us to identify not only cues about cleanliness and continence, but also about food and drinking habits, smoking and possibly physiological abnormalities such as dental caries or ketosis. Touch will tell us something about the patient's temperature, the condition of his skin, or the presence of irregularities in peripheral pulses. Using our ears will enable us to hear borborygmi or something about the patient's place of origin. It may also enable us to hear many things not expressed in words.

Aspects of Verbal and Non-verbal Communication

Some authorities say that as much as 90 per cent of interpersonal communication is non-verbal, and nurses must have knowledge of this area if useful information is not to be missed.

Although the term *non-verbal communication* refers to all the ways in which people receive and transmit information without the use of words, there are also non-verbal aspects of speech which transmit information and which are quite independent of the words being uttered. Indeed, it may be that the non-verbal cues are transmitting the opposite information to the words. For example, it is quite possible to say 'yes' in a tone of voice that indicates that we really mean 'no'. Again, someone who is upset may say 'I'm all right', while a shaky intonation indicates the opposite. In such situations, we tend to place greater reliance on the non-verbal than the verbal cues. It may be possible to correlate some aspects of speech with the patient's emotional state. For example, an anxious patient tends to talk faster than normal and at a higher pitch; an aggressive patient talks loudly. Disease may affect both the speed and delivery of speech.

In our culture, bodily contact is normally reserved to convey intimacy, aggression or a symbolic greeting in the form of a handshake or a pat on the back. However, in nursing, it may be necessary for proximity or social distance between patient and nurse to be reduced to the point of bodily contact to allow certain observations and nursing interventions to be made. It is usual that we indicate non-verbally that such close contact takes place on a professional rather than on a personal level.

Facial expressions can indicate a patient's emotional state. For example, we can learn to detect signs of happiness, surprise, fear, anger, disgust from facial expression. It is also possible to recognise degrees of emotional tension by perspiration on the forehead or palms of the hand, and dilatation of the pupils of the eyes.

Physical, Mental and Functional Assessment

We have already mentioned the desirability of making physical, mental and functional assessment, and our conviction that making them systematically will improve patient care. Some of the information will already be available in the medical notes and will therefore make asking questions about them again unnecessary. However, recording the information in the nursing history means that it, too can be taken into consideration when problems are identified. Sometimes this kind of information may do nothing more than direct our observations over the succeeding days or weeks, at others they will form the basis for action. Often they may be merely baseline information, allowing us to check whether an abnormality which we have just observed or to which our attention has been drawn was there previously or is a new development.

The list of observations which follows makes no claim to being complete. It should be seen merely as a guide to the kind of information which could be collected without difficulty. Different situations in which patients find themselves and different illnesses which may have brought them to hospital will require specific information.

Systems	*Observations*
Cardiovascular	Pulse – rate, rhythm, volume
	Blood pressure – lying, standing
	Venous pressure – height of pulsating jugular vein
	Skin colour – pale, flushed, cyanosed
Respiratory	Respirations – rate, depth, rhythm
	Dyspnoea, orthopnoea
	Cough – dry, productive
	Sputum – quantity, consistency, colour
	Accessory muscles of respiration used
	Barrel chest
Locomotor	General posture
	Paresis, paralysis
	Deformities – kyphosis, scoliosis, ulnar deviations
	Contractures
	Muscle wasting
Nervous	Level of consciousness
	Pupil size and reaction
	Pain – site, type
	Special senses – sight, hearing

Systems	Observations
Nervous (cont.)	Involuntary movement – tremor, choreiform or athetoid movements Dysphasia
Endocrine	Exophthalmos Polydypsia Enlarged thyroid Moon face Hyperactivity, underactivity
Gastrointestinal	Dentition Dysphagia Halitosis Nutritional state – obese, undernourished Constipation, diarrhoea
Genitourinary	Continence Discharges Pruritus Distended bladder Pregnancy
Integument	Personal hygiene Skin – bruising, abrasions, inflammation, hydration, pressure sores, purpura, pigmentation, temperature Nails – brittle, clubbed, koilonychia Hair – sparse, bald, infested

Mental state (mood adjectives)

Orientated, confused
Apprehensive, realistic
Anxious, friendly
Euphoric, aggressive
Depressed, withdrawn

Consideration of this list of adjectives should help us to give a fairly accurate description of the mental state of a patient during the assessment. It could also form a basis for indicating that a change has occurred over time.

A functional assessment is usually made informally. Observing the manner in which the patient enters the ward will give us quite a lot of information about his ability to function normally, as will observing the way he gets into his (high) hospital bed, his ability to hear our questions or read and complete his menu. Such information may affect nursing care directly. The patient may need two nurses to help him to the commode, or he may need to be addressed into his 'good' ear. It may also affect nursing care indirectly, by making us seek specialist help and advice on his behalf. What is important in either case is that our observations are written down so as to make them as accessible to the night nurse, or the nurse who arrives on the ward on the day the patient has his operation, as it was to us on admission.

Factors Which May Influence the Recording of Observations
A nursing history which has been recorded by one nurse will be available for reading by others who are to be involved in that patient's care. There is a great onus on the nurse, therefore, to record her observations objectively, accurately and precisely. If we are to make objective observations, then we need to be aware that we tend to notice what we desire to see, expect to see, have been trained to notice, or have been led to expect to see. We can however guard against our observations being influenced by such factors.

To record observations objectively entails that cues received through our sense organs be initially recorded without any attempt to interpret them. At this point it may be useful to say something about cues and inferences. We may, for example, see that a person has only scanty hair, hear that he speaks with a quavering voice, and feel that his skin is thin and inelastic. All these are cues. An inference, on the other hand, is a person's subjective interpretation or opinion based on a group of cues. In this case we may infer that the cues which we collected indicate that we are dealing with an old person. Scanty hairgrowth, a quavering voice, a dry and inelastic skin observed in isolation would not necessarily convey the same message to us, nor may establishing the patient's age by itself help us to decide whether or not he is his age, or 'young for his age'.

The first step to recording observations accurately therefore requires us to have a working knowledge of the difference between these two concepts, and practice at interviewing and also at analysing information contained in existing records may help to develop this. Asking oneself 'How did I know that?' may help us to identify just where our information came from.

To record observations accurately and precisely enables others who were not present when the history was being taken to share the experience vividly. Once cues have been noticed the ability to describe them will depend on our general as well as on our technical vocabulary. For example, a junior nurse with a limited professional vocabulary related to the cardiovascular system may record that a patient has a 'rapid pulse', whereas a senior nurse whose professional vocabulary is more extensive may record that the patient has 'a thready irregular pulse of 130'. This kind of precision and accuracy in recording observations may well affect the planning of that patient's nursing care.

General vocabulary can also be seen to influence the recording of observations. Feels well, not complaining, satisfactory at time of report, tell us little of importance about the patient. Has been free from pain since noon, able to walk to dayroom unaided, visit from wife has caused patient to be more cheerful are more informative as well as more accurate statements about the patient, and moreover can form the basis for future or ongoing assessment.

There is one other point which concerns collecting information from the patient. Looking carefully at what we have done to date, we may notice that we have got information from two sources – from what the patient told us and from what we ourselves observed. What the patient told us can be classified as subjective information, and is similar to what doctors refer to as symptoms. Objective information is based on the observations which we ourselves have made, and is similar to the signs of an illness which doctors collect. The status of these two types of information is different and will have to be used in different ways when we proceed to the next aspect of the nursing assessment – inspection of information and problem identification.

Inspection of Information and Problem Identification

Having recorded a nursing history we shall now be in possession of descriptive information about the patient and his situation. The final step in completing the first stage of the nursing process is to inspect the information to enable us to identify the patient's nursing problems. As we are dealing with a nursing history we would of course expect to identify only nursing problems. Let us take an example:

The doctor may identify that the patient's medical problem is carcinoma of the rectum requiring a permanent colostomy. The nurse, on the other hand, may identify that the same patient is extremely anxious about having his first ever anaesthetic, convinced that a colostomy will smell and thus make him socially unacceptable, and that he has grave doubts about his ability to cope with it.

There are two categories into which nursing problems may helpfully be divided. We may define patient problems as actual or potential problems. An actual patient problem is one that is present at a specific point in time and can be identified from the nursing history. A potential problem is one that has a high chance of occurring, but which can be influenced and possibly prevented or ameliorated by prescribed nursing action. These categories emphasise nurses' dual responsibility for curative and preventive nursing care.

We may also recall that the definition of health used at the beginning of this chapter suggested that a nursing history directed itself to three aspects of health, physical, mental and social. This is in keeping with the second method of categorising patient problems amenable to nursing care. Identifying a patient's emotional and social problems from a nursing history as well as his physical problems, and additionally deciding whether these problems are actual or potential demonstrates the concept of total patient care.

To assist us with the analysis of the information recorded in a patient's nursing history we have broken it down into five steps:

Checking that information is descriptive
Examining information for omissions and inconsistencies
Drawing inferences
Interpreting inferences to identify problems
Validating the existence of problems

Checking That Information Is Descriptive
Recording a nursing history is a purely descriptive process, so we would not expect to find any inferences contained in it. This

seems straightforward until we realise that people, including nurses, have a tendency to record their own interpretation or opinion of a situation rather than their actual observations. For example, we observe that the patient's hearing aid is on his locker, and may record that he dislikes wearing his hearing aid. However, one cue does not permit us to make an inference, and certainly not an accurate one, as there may be a number of reasons for the patient's hearing aid to be on the locker. For example it may be broken, the patient may want a rest, or he may have been unable to manipulate the hearing aid without assistance. Any information which is contained in a nursing history and which is not strictly factual (which may include what the patient said, though it may have been inaccurate) should therefore be treated with great caution.

Examining Information for Omissions and Inconsistencies
Before proceeding to drawing inferences from recorded cues, we need to examine the nursing history on two counts: first, for omissions and, second, for inconsistencies. To be admitted for a breast biopsy provokes anxiety in itself, but knowing that the patient's mother and grandmother died of breast cancer adds a new dimension to the amount of anxiety experienced. To avoid omissions we need to check that all possible sources of information have been searched, and no significant questions omitted.

Secondly, we examine the information for inconsistencies. A patient who says that he is not anxious about coming into hospital or about his impending operation may communicate the opposite non-verbally. Throughout the interview he may have had a high facial colour, sat on the edge of his chair, fiddled with his hands and even have been inarticulate at times, especially when conversation was about his operation. His pulse and blood pressure reading may have been raised. If inconsistencies are noted it is safer to assume that the patient has a problem in that area until and unless further information proves otherwise.

Drawing Inferences
For an inference to be accurate, it must be based on a group of cues, as relying on a single one may be insufficient and could lead to inaccuracy. To illustrate the difference between a cue

and an inference, and also how to draw an inference from a group
of cues we give some examples.

Cue	Inference
Bald	
Receding hair including eyebrows white	
Deep wrinkles in skin	
No teeth and sunken cheeks and lips	Elderly
History of bedrest	
Admitted in wheelchair	
Atrophy of calf muscles	
Has brought two walking sticks with him	Moves with difficulty
Does not know what day it is	
Tries to get into wrong bed	
Keeps asking where he is	
Cannot recall home address	Confused
Bed clothes wet when got out of bed	
Reddened sacral and genital areas	
Pool of water underneath chair after lunch	Difficulty in
Agitated when asked to wait for a bedpan	controlling micturition
No children	
Lives alone	
Retired	
Rehoused recently	
Does not know neighbours' names	Socially isolated

If we look at the first cue in each case we realise that no one
cue permits us to conclude that the individual was elderly, immobile,
confused, incontinent, or socially isolated. But if several cues are
taken together, they reinforce each other and allow an accurate
inference to be drawn.

Interpreting Inferences To Identify Problems
Having drawn inferences from cues recorded in a patient's nursing
history we now need to interpret their significance.

A single inference may constitute a problem for the patient
or be of no significance at all. For example, the inference of
elderly is of no significance in itself, whereas the inference of
incontinent constitutes an actual problem for the patient.

Once the significance of individual inferences has been decided, we need to analyse the significance of all the inferences drawn from the patient's nursing history. Interpreting the significance of a combination of inferences enables us to identify any actual or potential problems for that patient. Obviously, if we can identify such problems then prescribing nursing care can try to treat them or prevent them from becoming actual problems.

For example, if we look at the combination of inferences from a nursing history which indicates that the patient is elderly, incontinent, confused and immobile this would enable us to identify the need to deal with the incontinence, confusion and immobility as well as with his great potential for developing pressure sores. If we inferred that a patient was obese and immobile then we could identify his potential for developing deep vein thrombosis. A patient who was inferred to be blind and a smoker raises actual and potential problems of safety. If we have inferred that a patient is socially isolated and has now an added problem of being immobile, then we have to question whether he will be able to cope at home in future.

When we have interpreted the significance of combinations of inferences from the cues within the patient's nursing history, we will have a list of nursing problems. Some may be actual problems, some potential problems which may be mainly physical, emotional or social in nature.

Validating the Existence of Problems
What we have inferred to be a problem now has to be validated. This means that we need to return to the patient for confirmation of the fact that a particular problem does exist. Techniques of validating may be described as either objective or subjective validation of problems. We are already familiar with these terms from the earlier part of this chapter.

If a nurse has made an inference that a patient has abdominal pain, she may return to the patient to validate objectively whether the problem does exist. This may be done by observing the patient for cues such as facial grimaces, tachycardia, hands clutching the painful area, knees drawn up to chest or the like.

To validate subjectively whether the patient has abdominal pain again requires the nurse to return to the patient but this time she would ask him whether he had a pain.

In this example, the observations of the nurse (objective validation) and the opinion of the patient (subjective validation) tallied
and together confirmed the existence of the patient's problem of
pain. This may seem fairly obvious, but there may be occasions
when the nurse has to rely purely on validating the existence
of a patient's problem objectively. Such occasions may occur when
dealing with the confused, the unconscious or the very young.

Even when dealing with patients who can participate in validating
the existence of a problem, there will be occasions when we rely
more on our own observations than on the patient's opinion. For
example, we may have inferred that a man who has recently had
a myocardial infarction, who is a heavy smoker, obese and a piece-
worker on a building site has a potential problem of adapting his
lifestyle to suit his health requirements. He has been advised about
the need for reducing weight, stopping smoking and restricting
his previous schedule of activity. When objectively validating
whether the problem exists we observe that the patient is openly
smoking, regularly deviating from his diet, and engaging in more
exercise than he is supposed to do. Our observations confirm the
existence of the inferred problem.

However, on subjectively validating the existence of the problem
the patient says that he feels almost 100 per cent again, and that
the doctor must have exaggerated the severity of the heart attack.

The fact that we made an inference about a problem not only
objectively but also subjectively validates its existence in spite
of what the patient says, and in addition gives the patient another
opportunity to acknowledge rather than deny that the problem
exists.

When we approach the patient to validate subjectively the existence of a problem we need to be aware that the rather shy
patient may be reticent about disagreeing with us. Such patients
will need the encouragement of a question such as 'Have I got
it right?' or 'Am I correct in thinking?' to allow him to express
his true opinion about the existence or otherwise of a problem.

The technique of subjectively validating the existence of a problem encourages patient involvement. This seems the logical thing
to do when we consider that we are dealing with patient problems
and not nurse problems. If the patient can be helped to recognise

the problem he has, or may have in the future, as a result of his illness, he can participate in suggesting solutions to solve or minimise his problem. This is important when we realise that solutions suggested by the person who has the problem are usually considered more relevant than suggestions imposed on them by others.

Writing Problem Statements

Having identified nursing problems we now have to commit them to paper. Writing problem statements can take two forms. There is first the multiple problem approach, where each individual problem that has been identified is written down separately. For example, we can say that the patient needs help with washing, feeding, toileting. Alternatively, there is the central problem approach. This means that when there is a common denominator to a patient's problems this unifying theme can shape all the nursing care the patient receives, with individual problems subsumed under it. To take the previous example, we might state that the patient needs help with carrying out activities of daily living.

Problem statements should be written as precisely as the information allows. Stereotyped problem statements such as pain, anxiety, constipation are lacking in precision. Several patients in a ward may have these problems but as the cause may be different in each case so may the required nursing action. This means that the level of precision of the written problem statement should be such as to allow us to plan appropriate nursing care.

Problem statements should also be concise. They should contain no unnecessary words and in some instances the use of commonly accepted abbreviations and symbols may be permissible.

Summary

We have established that the assessment stage of the nursing process involves two distinct acts: firstly, the collection of objective and subjective information in the form of observable cues; secondly, the analysis of such cues. This involves drawing inferences from the observed cues, interpreting the significance of inferences to enable us to identify both actual and potential problems, which may be of a physical, emotional or social nature. By validating the existence of problems objectively and subjectively we are equipped to proceed to the second stage of the nursing process, that of planning personalised nursing care.

To help us decide who should carry out the assessment stage of the nursing process we need to be guided by two considerations. First, the four stages of the process are interrelated, with assessment forming the foundation. Therefore a care plan can only be as good as the assessment on which it is based. Second, to be proficient at collecting and assessing information requires many skills. All

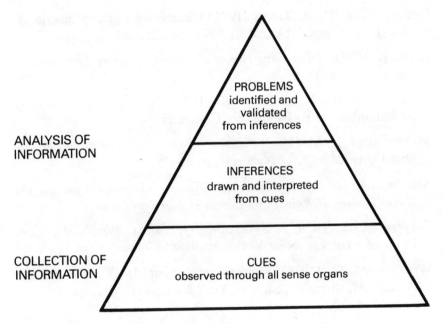

Fig. 2. Outline of problem identification based on assessment.

nurses will initially be students of the nursing process, but the qualified nurse with her knowledge and previous experience is likely to become proficient more quickly at assessment than will the student nurse. Considering that the more experienced nurse may be the more appropriate one to carry out assessment is in contrast to the present system where the most junior nurse, or the ward clerk, is often thought capable of admitting a patient.

The nursing process requires us to acknowledge the importance of collecting and analysing base-line information about every new patient, and in this way provide quality individualised patient care.

References and Suggested Further Readings

Abercrombie, J. (1968) *The Anatomy of Judgement*. Harmondsworth: Penguin.

Argyle, M. (1973) *The Psychology of Interpersonal Behaviour*. London: Pelican.

Bircher, A. V. (1975) On the development and classification of diagnoses. *Nursing Forum*, Vol. 14, No. 1, pp. 11–29.

Gebbie, K. & M. A. Lavin (1974) Classifying nursing diagnoses. *Am. J. of Nursing* (February, 1974) pp. 250–53.

Crow, J. (1978) *The Nursing Process*. London: *Nursing Times* Publication.

Little, D. E. & D. L. Carnevali (1976) *Nursing Care Planning*. Philadelphia: J. B. Lippincott Company.

McPhetridge, L. M. (1968) Nursing history: one means to personalised care. *Am. J. of Nursing*, pp. 68–75.

Macilwaine, H. (1977) *Teaching Effective Communication in the Nurse/Patient Relationship*. London: *Nursing Times*.

Mayers, M. A. (1978) *A Systematic Approach to the Nursing Care Plan*. 2nd edition. New York: Appleton-Century-Crofts.

Wolanin, M. O. (1976) Nursing assessment. In *Nursing and the Aged*, I. M. Burnside, ed. New York & London: McGraw-Hill, pp. 398–420.

3. Planning Nursing Care

The type of information required in assessment enables us to identify patients' problems so that we can plan care.

The planning of nursing care is an essential step before carrying out the activity of nursing the patient. Planning is of particular importance in this age of technological care to ensure that the nursing care is consciously directed towards alleviating the patients' problems and meeting their needs. To omit the planning stage may result in the nursing care being focussed on the technical aspects of the patient's care at the expense of caring for the patient as a person and meeting all his problems.

It is the giving of this personal care, which is planned to meet a patient's particular problems, that ensures the most effective nursing care for each patient. Without careful planning nursing care will be disorganised and less effective.

Steps in Planning Nursing Care

Planning the patient's care involves four steps:

1. Determining priorities. This involves analysing the problems identified in the assessment stage to decide which problems require priority of attention.

2. Setting goals. These state what is to be achieved if the identified problems are to be alleviated.

3 Selecting nursing actions. This involves choosing the methods and techniques which will enable us to achieve the stated patient goals.

4. Writing the care plan. The problems, goals and nursing actions are recorded on the patient's nursing care plan.

The steps involved in planning care are illustrated using some of the problems identified from the nursing assessment of Mr Watney (see pp. 63–68).

Determining Priorities

The first step is to decide which of the identified problems must be dealt with immediately. What are the problems which require immediate attention? There are two types: those which are life-threatening and those which impinge on the safety of the patient.

The assessment of Mr Watney reveals the following life-threatening problem:

> Inadequate pulmonary ventilation resulting in poor perfusion of the tissues with oxygen.

This problem will be a priority for both the nursing care and the medical treatment. It will have been identified from the information given to the nurse by the admitting doctor. The nurse will provisionally plan the patient's care in relation to this problem by ensuring that oxygen, face mask and other essentials are at the bedside ready for the patient's arrival. When the patient arrives the nurse initiates immediate nursing action to deal with the problem by following the doctor's instructions of administering oxygen. Having planned and instituted nursing care to deal with this life-threatening problem we can turn our attention to planning care for other non-life-threatening problems. However, the problem related to inadequate pulmonary ventilation will remain a priority in importance even though it may no longer be life-threatening as a result of the immediate action taken.

The remaining problems may appear to be of equal importance. However, not all can be dealt with at once. There has to be some further ordering of priorities. What importance we place on the problem will be influenced by the importance the patient attaches to it. If the patient is very concerned about one particular problem this may well influence his recovery and reaction to the nursing care he is receiving. Nursing care directed to another problem at the expense of the one considered most important by the patient will be less effective. This is because the patient reacts *totally* to a situation in which his problem is not considered important by the nursing staff.

The assessment of Mr Watney reveals other problems, for example:

1. Inadequate understanding of his illness and how he acquired this chest infection.
2. Concern about his wife's management of their finances.

Our priority may be to deal with the patient's inadequate knowledge of his present condition and to leave dealing with the problem related to his wife and money to the social worker at a later date. However, any attempt to teach the patient about his chest condition will be negated by the patient's concern over the problem of money. He will interpret our nursing action of dealing with the other problem first as indicating that the money problem is of little concern to us. However, if our nursing plan initiates action in relation to the money problem, for example, asking the medical social worker to talk to Mr Watney and his wife, then he will feel that the necessary steps are being taken to deal with what he considers to be the most important problem. He will, as a result, be more receptive to our nursing intervention related to the problem of education, which he himself considers to be of less importance.

With each problem that we identify we have to decide whether it is directly or indirectly amenable to nursing action. For example, Mr Watney's problem related to money is not directly amenable to nursing intervention, as it lies outside our sphere of expertise. It is, however, indirectly amenable to nursing action in that it is our responsibility to refer the problem to the medical social worker – the appropriate source of help. Similarly, a patient developing atrial fibrillation following a myocardial infarction requires medical intervention. The indirect nursing intervention consists of recognising this condition, taking the appropriate action of calling the doctor, and monitoring the condition of the patient.

Setting Goals
Whenever a problem is identified there is an implication that the present situation is unsatisfactory for the patient or the nurse or both. If this were not so then there would be no need for the patient to accept our help or for us to offer it.

Patients may use a variety of words when expressing their personal goals; for example, they may talk of their hopes, desires, aims, wants or wishes. Whatever term is used by the patient the words indicate a change from the present situation to one that is more desirable.

To help the patient with the identified problems we must know what is to be achieved. Knowledge of *what* is to be achieved is necessary before we can decide *how* it is to be achieved. It also enables us to measure the effect of our nursing care in terms of changes in the patient's condition indicating progress towards the desired outcome, solving the problem.

Characteristics of goals for nursing care
The goal must indicate *what* changes are to take place in the patient's behaviour or condition as a result of our nursing care; that is, it gives direction to our care. It must also state *how* the expected changes in the patient's behaviour or condition will be observed and indicate *when* he is expected to have achieved it.

A useful goal is realistic. It must be possible for the patient to achieve what the goal states as the desirable outcome. If goals are unrealistic the patient may become disillusioned because he is not progressing at the speed he expected, or it may lead him to think that he is able to do more than he actually is capable of. It would be unrealistic to expect a patient following a stroke to achieve full mobility if he had a considerable degree of residual paralysis. More realistic goals should be stated which indicate that he would adapt his activities to make his limited mobility less of a problem.

The focus of the goal would, therefore, be to help the patient to make more effective use of his functioning limbs, or to modify his daily activities and lifestyle to cope with his residual paralysis, if necessary with assistance from someone else – a relative, friend or a nurse. The over-all aim is to allow the patient to function adequately and as independently as possible in his environment.

The factors to be considered when setting goals for nursing care are:

a. Goals must be patient-centred.
b. Goals must be concisely stated.
c. Action verbs must be used in the statement of the goal.

d. The type of behaviour expected from the patient must be qualified.

e. A time element must be included.

Set patient-centred goals
The problems that we have identified are those experienced by the patient. It follows, therefore, that the goals should state the changes to be expected as a result of the patient's behaviour, and not the nurse's behaviour. A goal that starts with the words 'assist, enable, permit or encourage the patient to . . .' is stated in terms of what the nurse will be doing and not how the patient will behave. For example, 'Encourage the patient to drink extra fluids' states the nurse's behaviour and not the patient's.

A patient-centred goal would be 'Increase fluid intake from 1½ litres in twenty-four hours to 2½ litres in twenty-four hours', or 'drink one glass of orange squash each hour during the daytime'.

State goal concisely
The previous patient-centred example illustrates a concisely stated goal. If we always state patient-centred goals it is unnecessary to commence each statement with the phrase 'The patient will', as this is implicit. By omitting this phrase the goal is not only more concise, but it also allows us to commence the statement with an action verb, which gives the statement greater impact.

Use action verbs
Commencing the statement with an action verb focusses our attention on the behaviour which our nursing actions will enable the patient to achieve. It also indicates what we need to observe to evaluate whether the patient has reached the goal.

In the example the action verb *increase* or *drink* indicates immediately what is to be achieved and what is to be observed, that is, an increase, to indicate that the goal has been achieved.

Qualify the patient's behaviour
Apart from the action associated with the goal it may be necessary to state the manner in which that action is to be carried out; for example, 'negotiate stairs *safely*', 'dress *independently*', or 'speak *coherently*'. These qualifying words give the goal more precision.

Identify a time element

It may be important for goals to be met within a certain time, for example, before discharge, before theatre, before transfer to another unit, or before treatment can commence. The time element in the example about fluid intake is precisely stated. The goal indicates not only how much fluid has to be taken, but also states the period of time over which the increase in fluid intake is to be achieved.

Some goals deal with changes that take a long time to achieve. With our stroke patient one goal may be that he should 'Get out of bed and dress independently before discharge'. It may be a while before the patient is able to carry out the activities stated in the goal. As a result both the patient and the nurse may become disheartened.

What is needed is for this long-term goal to be broken down into short-term goals. The patient is then helped to achieve each of these short-term goals. They are introduced to him one at a time so that he can concentrate on each one until he achieves the desired outcome.

The long-term goal 'Get out of bed and dress independently before discharge' could involve the following short-term goals:

1. Get out of bed onto bedside chair with assistance.
2. Get out of bed onto bedside chair independently.
3. Put trousers on while sitting on chair, with assistance.
4. Put trousers on while standing, with assistance.
5. Put trousers on while standing, without assistance.
6. Put shirt on independently, with assistance in fastening buttons.
7. Fasten buttons on shirt alone, with assistance only for buttons on cuff of non-paralysed arm.

The achievement of each of these goals contributes to the long-term goal of being able to get out of bed and dress independently. Because both the patient and we ourselves are experiencing frequent success in achieving these short-term goals neither of us is likely to become disheartened. We can offer the patient praise and feel a measure of success for our own hard work, while our patient can feel a sense of achievement and progress on his long struggle to independence.

Selecting Nursing Actions To Meet Goals

One problem experienced by Mr Watney which we identified was:

Inadequate pulmonary ventilation resulting in poor perfusion of the tissues with oxygen.

A nursing care goal in relation to this problem might be stated as:

Increased intake of oxygen at each respiratory effort, bringing about improvement in perfusion of the tissues with oxygen indicated by the respiratory function test in twenty-four hours time.

The achievement of this goal will involve consideration of these aspects of nursing care:

1. Providing an oxygen-enriched atmosphere.
2. Ensuring that the patient adopts a position and posture that will maximise pulmonary ventilation at each inspiratory effort.
3. Administering drugs prescribed by the doctor which will further increase effective pulmonary ventilation.
4. Facilitating the expectoration of retained sputum.

One factor influencing the choice of nursing actions will be the doctor's instructions. These instructions will usually be related to the life-threatening problems and may, therefore, often assume priority. However, nursing intervention related to the doctor's instructions must not only ensure that these are carried out but be done in a manner to help the patient through the experience by explanations and concern for him as a person.

The nursing care for Mr Watney which is determined by the doctor's instructions is the administration of oxygen. The doctor has prescribed that it should be given at a concentration of 28 per cent via a Venturi mask. However, there are other nursing actions associated with the administration of oxygen that are independent of the doctor's instructions. For example, we will explain to Mr Watney why oxygen is being administered and how it will help him. This will assist him in realising the importance of keeping the mask in place. We will also try to minimize the discomfort which the elastic on the mask may cause him. This would be achieved by placing a piece of gauze beneath the elastic where it causes pain due to pressure, for example, above his ears. We will also ensure that the safety precautions are observed to reduce the risk of fire when oxygen is being administered.

The choice of the nursing actions may also be influenced by the policies of the hospital. The nursing assessment of Mr Watney reveals that he normally takes a snack at bedtime before retiring. Hospital policy may be to serve the last food to patients at 6:30 P.M. and to provide only a drink prior to retiring. The nursing action to meet Mr Watney's need in this situation might be to ask him to save part of his evening meal, for example, his cheese and biscuits, until bedtime, or to get his wife to bring him sandwiches at visiting time, if alternative arrangements to provide a late snack cannot be made.

Each goal may be achieved by one of several nursing actions. The choice is determined by our knowledge of which is the most appropriate action for the individual patient.

Our knowledge and creativity will determine the range of alternatives from which we may choose and our ability to offer unique solutions to unique problems. The selection of the appropriate action is not only dependent on our knowledge and creativity but directly related to our knowledge of the individual patient and the correct identification of his problems.

The choice of the nursing actions is communicated to the patient and its acceptability to him is noted and taken into account. However, there are times when our decisions must overrule the patient's preferences. This must be done in such a manner that the patient feels that he still retains some control over what happens to him. The patient may be involved in deciding which is the most appropriate action to take. For example, it may be desirable to increase Mr Watney's fluid intake. This goal is more likely to be achieved if we give him a choice of which fluid he would prefer to drink, rather than just telling him to drink more water, which he may dislike. The involvement of the patient in the decision-making process helps him to realise that he is an active participant in his own care, not just a passive receiver of nursing care.

In addition to deciding on the nursing actions we must also decide how and when we will measure the patient's progress towards achieving the goal. For example, we may decide to take peak-flow measurements on Mr Watney every four hours. These will indicate the effectiveness of the nursing care (and medical treatment) in achieving the goal of 'improved pulmonary ventilation'.

Recording Information on the Nursing Care Plan

The nursing actions, the method and time of evaluation are written on the patient's care plan alongside the statement of the problem and the goal. Writing down this information forces us to return to our plans at frequent intervals, partly to ensure that we are doing what we planned to do, and also to indicate if our goals have been met. In other words, plans *must* be used and not just completed and then filed away. Care plans are only useful if they are kept up-to-date.

This discussion has used certain problems from Mr Watney's nursing assessment to take us through the steps involved in planning patient care. We have:

Stated the problem
Set goals
Determined nursing actions, and
Stated how and when progress should be evaluated

Nursing Care Plans

The examples of completed care plans illustrate how the nursing care plan is derived from the accompanying nursing histories and assessments.

In example 1 we have used two different history formats to demonstrate that, provided they are used carefully, they will allow us to identify the same problems.

The entries under 'Evaluation' may be said to constitute only short-term and interim evaluations (or even reassessments), or they might, perhaps, even be seen as further nursing activities. Whatever view we take, there is no doubt that a more comprehensive evaluation will be necessary before we are in a position to decide that the tissues, for example, are now adequately perfused with oxygen, and therefore problem no. 1 has been resolved.

The second nursing history and care plan (example 2) highlight two important points. Firstly, by setting the completed nursing history and the information which was actually recorded in the Kardex side by side, we clearly demonstrate how the extra information in the nursing history was used to identify the patient's problems enabling personalised nursing care to be given. Without taking such a history a number of problems would not have been identified.

This nursing history uses a structured and semistructured format and was compiled specifically to assess the needs of the injured elderly. It was found helpful to use a more structured format as it offered greater direction. Having become familiar with this detailed nursing history a nurse would be able to use a semistructured or an unstructured format with only headings to act as a reminder to areas to be investigated.

The care plan illustrates the total care the patient received from admission to transfer home. In addition it was possible to accompany the district nurse on her first visit to the patient, and to see the patient when she attended outpatients for her first follow-up appointment, which is reflected in the continuation of the care plan after the patient was transferred to the community nursing staff. (This nursing history and care plan were first published in *Nursing Times* and are reproduced with permission.)

The last nursing history and care plan (example 3) originated in a children's ward. They illustrate a situation where it was necessary to include the patient along with her carer in the assessment phase as well as in planning for and giving nursing care. It contains a large teaching component and shows that only dealing with the problems displayed by the patient would have been unlikely to have resulted in meeting her problems adequately.

History and Care Plans Examples

1. James Watney

2. Doris Adams

3. Julie Bea

Nursing History Sheet   Hospital no. *A52304*   Surname *Watney*   First names *James*

Ward   Date of birth *14/1/1926*   Age *53*   Religion *Baptist*

Social History

Occupation *None - retired because of chest condition*

Marital state *Married*

Children *1*   Ages *22*

Do you live alone? *No*

Any aged or young dependants *Son lives and works away at present*

Next-of-kin *Wife*

Relationship

Home telephone no. *None*

Office telephone no. *None*

Neighbour's telephone no. *—*

Distance for visiting *5 miles*

Hobbies/Interests *Reading westerns, watching television*

Would you like to see the Hospital Chaplain? *Yes, if he visits*

Any language barrier or speech defect *None although he has difficulty with long words*

Previous Hospitalization

Where? *Here*

When? *Each year, in winter over last 7 – 8 years*

Health Problems

Diabetes *—*

Heart disease *—*

Asthma *—*

Epilepsy *—*

Enuresis *—*

Any other *Chronic bronchitis*

Admission Information

Date *5 August 1979*

Time *10 a.m.*

Mode *Ambulance*

Accompanied by *Wife*

From where? *Home*

Dr's explanation to patient for this admission *To treat chest infection*

Recent colds, infections etc *Contact with friend who had flu*

Diet

No. of meals a day *Breakfast, lunch and evening meal. Prefer snack at bedtime*

Special diet *—*

Fluid preferences *Dislikes milky drinks*

Allergies *None*

Sleep *Retires late, sleeps in at morning until 10 a.m.*

Normal sleep pattern

Daytime naps? *None*

Sedation taken *None*

If unable to sleep, what else helps? *Cup of tea*

Pain

Has patient any pain? *No*

Where? *—*

What type? *—*

Elimination

Urinary: Frequency *Every 4 – 5 hours*

Incontinent *No*

Dysuria *None*

Nocturia *None*

Bowel Movements: Daily *Yes, first thing in morning*

Other *—*

Type of laxative taken *Senokot, if needed*

How often? *Only if constipated*

Remarks

Name Mr T. Watney
Nursing History Sheet

Drugs

Currently using Franol
How often 8 hourly
Spinhaler - every 4 hours

General appearance
Normal Slouches down in bed, stoops when standing
Obese
Thin Looks thin, but is quite tall
Emaciated

General condition
Comfortable/(Anxious)/Distressed
V. distressed/ orientated (Responsive)
Not fully responsive/Unresponsive

Hearing
(Good)/poor/wears aid No

Vision
(Good)/poor/wears glasses No
Always/Reading only
Prosthesis
What type? None
Help needed?

Oral hygiene
Condition of mouth Dry and slight white coating
Condition of teeth Good
Have you dentures? No

Skin
Dehydrated No
Oedematous Slight ankle oedema
Broken areas Redness over sacral area on both sides
Other

Mobility
Bathing Self, when not dyspnoeic
Dressing Self
Feeding Self
Toileting Commode or sanichair to toilet
Walking Short distances, then becomes dyspnoeic
Remarks Normally able to walk to shops at own pace
General observations
T 38°C P 98 R 28 BP 130/70
Height 185cm (6'1") Weight 64 kg (140 lbs)
Urine Routine ward test - no abnormalities

Additional significant observations
made while taking history
Says he has been admitted because he caught 'flu from a friend.
Dislikes being cared for when ill.
Coughing up thick tenacious sputum yellow/green.
Concerned about wife - says she spends too much money.
Not very knowledgeable about his condition and reason for chest infection.
Significant details of medical care
Tidal vol = 400 ml $PaO_2 = 61$ mmHg
$PaCO_2 = 49$ mmHg
To have antibiotics and oxygen 28%

History obtained from Patient
If not a patient, relationship to patient
Obtained by
Date 5/8/79
Time

Name **Mr Watney**

Age **53**

Nursing Assessment

Date **5/8/79**

Religion **Baptist**

Employment

Diagnosis **Chronic bronchitis with acute chest infection**

Patients interpretation of present illness

Not sure why he's in hospital, realises that he has got a chest infection but does not know how this came about

Drugs Franol - 2x3 times/day
Spinhaler spray

Allergies None

Elimination and sleep habits

Bowels usually opened daily, early morning. Takes Senokot occasionally if constipated. No difficulty with passing urine - does not get up at/night. Retires late, prefers to watch T.V. until late. Gets up about 10am.

Physical limitation

Can do most things for himself. Gets breathless if exerts himself excessively. Sight and hearing both good - does not wear spectacles. Dentures not worn.

Observations made during interview

A tall thin man, clean but untidy. Tends to slump down in bed or chair. Talks quietly, appears anxious when talking. Initiates conversation only occasionally. Alert and oriented. No signs of pain or discomfort.
Respirations - shallow and rapid   T. 38
No cyanosis   P. 98
Mouth dry - breathes   R. 28
through mouth   B/P. 130/70
Coughing up thick   Ht. 185 cm
tenacious sputum   Wt. 64 kg

Experience with previous illness

Admitted frequently over last 10 years; usually each winter.
Says he dislikes 'being cared for' when in hospital

Diet and food habits

Normally eats a normal diet - good appetite. Light breakfast, lunch and evening meal. Likes a snack at bedtimes. Dislikes milky drinks

Personal habits

No exercise taken, tends to sit in chair for most of the day. Likes watching T.V. & reading westerns. Does not go to church - but would like to talk to vicar if he visits.

Social history

Left school at 15, worked as a labourer, bar tender. Lives with wife and son in council semi, clean and not damp. Wife (45 years) works in factory locally - able to visit easily. Son - working away at present.

Concerns expressed by patient during interview

Worried that wife spends money irresponsibly - too much spent on food. Feels that his pension (disablement) does not contribute much to the family income.

Relevant details from medical notes.

Tidal vol   400 m
PaO_2 61 mm. Hg
$PaCO_2$ 49 mm Hg
HCO_3 30 mmol/litre

Name: Mr Watney

Problem	Goal	Nursing Care	Evaluation / reassessment
1. Inadequate pulmonary ventilation resulting in poor perfusion of the tissues with oxygen.	1. Increased intake of oxygen and/or inspiratory effort resulting in improved perfusion of the tissues with oxygen.	1. Administer oxygen at 4 litres/minute via 28% venturi mask and humidifier. 2. Correct patient's posture - sit upright supported with pillows. If he slides down or slouches in bed or chair remind him of importance of correct posture 3. Give moist inhalations as per Kardex, and get patient to cough and expectorate sputum. 4. Daily fluid intake to be at least 2 litres in 24 hours, no milky drinks. 5. Administer Spinhaler 6 hourly as per medicine Kardex	1. Check flow rate hourly 2. Top up humidifier 3. Patient will keep mask in place continually 4. Check patient's position in bed each time you enter room. 5. Record peak flow reading every 4 hours and chart. 6. Check that patient drinks at least 150 mls each hour, no milky drinks. 7. Observe colour and record amount of sputum expectorate every 12 hours.

Name **Mr J. Watney**

Problem	Goal	Nursing Care	Evaluation / reassessment
2. Possible development of pressure sores on buttocks.	2. Redness will disappear and no tissue breakdown will occur.	1. When in bed i. assist to turn to alternate sides every two hours (even hours 6, 8, 10 etc.) ii. patient to lift his buttocks clear of mattress for few seconds every two hours (odd hours 7, 9, 11 etc.) iii. sit on sheepskin when in bed or out in chair. 2. When in chair stand up and walk a few paces every two hours, assist if needed or requested. 3. Implement measures related to increasing perfusion of tissues with oxygen (problem 1)	1. Assess amount of redness over pressure area 6am, 12md. and 6pm. Record in Kardex. Report immediately to nurse in charge if redness increases or other discoloration occurs.
3. Inadequate knowledge about present condition and avoidance of chest infections	3. Increased knowledge about source of infection and measures to avoid chest infections	1. Talk with Mr Watney to ascertain just what he understands about why he keeps getting chest infections each year. 2. Explain need to avoid people with colds, and why he should avoid crowded public places especially in winter. 3. Explain advantages to him of having 'flu' vaccine each year.	1. When asked Mr Watney will be able to list the possible sources of infection and explain what steps he intends to take to avoid them. 2. He will express willingness to have the 'flu' vaccine.

Name Mr J. Watney

Problem	Goal	Nursing Care	Evaluation / reassessment
4. Nursing care threatens his feelings of independence.	4. Perform those activities which he is able to do with minimum assistance from the nurse....	1. Allow him to wash, bath, etc. unaided unless he asks for assistance or he becomes breathless. 2. When assisting him ask him the best way to help, or ascertain how he normally performs the task and follow his instructions	1. Mr Watney will express his willingness to let the nurses help him when he is unable to do things for himself.

Personal data

Name *Mrs Doris Adams*

Address *15 Alvis Close, Sheffield*

Date of birth *3/7/1893*   Age *82 years*

Source of admission *Emergency*

Hospital no. *BA 7908*

Date of injury *9/6/76*   Time *3.00pm*

Date of admission *9/6/76*   Time *7.00pm*

Reason for time lapse

Medical diagnosis *Fractured neck of (R) femur*

Previous hospital admission with reason,

date, hospital

1. Jessops, Lincoln, - Prolapse 1961

Do you remember anything in particular

about your stay? *Dr. asking personal questions so loudly the whole ward could hear*

Orientation programme required? *Yes*

If history not taken from the patient,

give reason, person's name and relationship

Patient's perception and expectations

about his/her injury

1. Why have you come to hospital?
I have broken my thigh. GP ordered ambulance to bring me.

2. What caused your injury?
Fell off third rung of stepladder while cutting hedge

3. What is your health normally like?
Good

4. Has anyone explained your injury and

   expected treatment to you?

They have told my son

5. What do you understand from their

   explanation?
I have broken my thigh and it needs a screw.

6. Is there anything you are anxious

   about regarding your injury or

   treatment? *Worried about my facial hair - my daughter usually sees to it.*

7. How long do you expect to be in hospital?
Two weeks

8. How do you expect to get on following

   discharge? *Hope to be all right, and no trouble to anyone.*

Physical/Safety data relating to daily

living activities

Pain

1. Have you any pain?

   Describe *Yes - but only when I move*

2. Did you have any pain before your

   injury? Describe
No.

3. What do you do to relieve this pain?

Sleep

1. Usual bedtime? *10.30 pm or later*

2. Hours of sleep per night? *Rise about 8.00 am*

3. Do you need to get up in the night?
Two to three times per night

4. Nap habits *No - do not need them*

5. Number of pillows? *Two*

6. If unable to sleep what do you do?
Just lie there - doesn't bother me.

7. Height of bed
Single divan

Hygiene

1. What facilities do you have for washing at home? *Bathroom - upstairs*

2. What facilities are you able to make use of? *Have a non-slip mat for the bath - my daughter just helps me in and out.*

3. Do you have dentures or your own teeth? *Own teeth*

4. If dentures, full top bottom partial?

5. Condition of dentures/teeth? *Poor - been to a dentist twice only*

6. How do you care for your dentures/teeth? *Toothbrush and paste*

7. Are you limited as to what you can eat due to your teeth? *No.*

8. What kind of skin do you have? *Good. (Pressure area care explained)*

Continence

1. What are your usual bowel habits?

   Frequency *Daily*   Time *a.m.*

2. Do you have any bowel irregularities? *Sometimes constipated*

3. What do you do for these irregularities? *Take a glass of Andrews - that is all that is needed*

4. Location of toilet *Just outside the back door - it is a bit cold on winter nights*

5. Usual bladder habits.

   Frequency *Varies*   Time *Nocte 2/3 times*

6. Do you have any trouble with your water? Describe *Burns sometimes, and sometimes incontinent.*

7. Are you worried about these functions while in hospital? *Bothered about being a burden as normally manage my incontinence without any trouble to my daughter.*

Feeding

Food

1. Were you on a special diet before admission? *No.*

2. Did you have any problems with this diet or in preparing meals? *No. Cooked a hot meal every evening for her daughter and herself.*

3. Usual meal patterns   Time   Usual Foods

   Breakfast *8.00 am* *Toast and marmalade*
   Lunch   *1.00 pm* *Cheese sandwich*
   Dinner   *6.00 pm* *Meat and 2 vegetables*
   Snacks   *Milk and biscuit at 11.00 and before bedtime*

Drinks

1. Amount drunk normally in a day? *About 2 litres/day*

2. Type of fluids? *Tea and milk*

3. Fluid preferences? *Horlicks, but too expensive - now have extra milk instead.*

4. Fluid dislikes? *Not keen on coffee.*

Ambulation and safety factors

1. Do you normally have any difficulty walking? *No*

2. Do you envisage difficulty walking when you go home? *No*

3. Do you use any walking aids? *No*

4. Do you have difficulty manipulating items, eg dressing?
Back zip on dresses only - daughter helps then

5. Do you have difficulty with seeing?
Wears glass all day .

6. Do you have difficulty with hearing?
Wears hearing aid , NHS and private Both are in hospital with her

7. Do you smoke?
No.

Assessment of patient's capabilities

By patient before injury-

Ambulation *Independent, fully mobile*

Feeding *Independent*

Bathing *Independent*

Elimination *Some incontinence*

Special care *Nil*

By nurse on admission

Ambulation *Immobile*

Feeding *Needs assistance*

Bathing *Needs assistance*

Elimination *Requires bedpans*

Special care *To traction*

Joint assessment by patient/nurse before discharge

Ambulation *Independent with frame , and can manage stairs*

Feeding *Independent*

Bathing *Independent washing at sink . Independent at dressing*

Elimination *Independent, incontinence rectified*

Special care
Requires dressing to hip wound

Social/Interpersonal data

Family

1. Name and address of next-of-kin?
Miss Doris Adams, same address as patient

2. Has she been informed/do you wish her to be informed?
Is with patient while history being recorded

3. Do you mind my discussing your injury with her? *No.*

4. Has your being admitted made any difference to her life?
I normally cook all the meals for when she comes home from work

5. Composition of family
I daughter single I son married

6. What are their ages?
56 years and 50 years

7. What are their occupations?
Typist, and son works in a moulding shop

8. What is their health like?
Daughter has sinus and back trouble .

9. How often do you see your family?
Son fetches me and my daughter at 5.00pm every Sat. and we are home by 19.00 pm

10. How far away do they live?
Son lives half-hour car ride away.

11. Do you help each other in any way?
My son's child who is now married used to help. My daughter and I help each other.

12. Do you expect them to visit?
Yes.

13. Does anyone have a key to your house?

Son and daughter

14. If alone, are you worried about pets,

cancelling orders, water pipes,

paying the rent etc?

Occupation

1. Your past/present occupation?

Before being married was a 'saw screw and nut finisher' – attached the handle to saws. Cleaner for 8yrs after husband died – 3 floors for 3d.

2. Did you have many jobs? *Only 2*

3. What do you enjoy doing now?

Watching colour T.V., gardening and cooking

Housing

1. What sort of area-industrial,

residential etc? *Residential*

2. Are you on a bus route? *Yes*

3. Are you able to use the buses?

Odd times – 2yrs since last went to town.

4. How far away is the nearest shop? *200yd*

5. Do you do your own shopping and

housework? *My daughter and I share it*

6. Council property or private ownership?

Council property

7. Are most of your neighbours your age?

Most are retired.

8. How well do you know them?

Well – lived there over 20yrs.

9. Describe your accommodation

2-bedroomed town-house

10. Does the layout of your house present

any problems? *No- but had thought about buying a commode for use at night, but cost £16.*

11. What heating/cooking facilities do

you have?

Immersion heater, gas cooker and fire, electric blanket.

Spiritual need

1. What religion are you? *Church of England*

2. Do you normally attend Church?

No- used to do years ago.

3. Do you wish your own minister to be

informed? *I don't know his name*

4. Are you aware the hospital chaplain

visits all patients routinely and

is available any time patients wish

to see him? *Yes, he has had a word with me already; he came to see some other lady in the ward, not especially me.*

Community care data

1. When did you last see your GP and

for what? *Saw him today before my fall. It was 6 months before that with headaches; he gave me just one course of tablets.*

2. Medications

1. *None*

2.

3.

Disposition: home   pharmacy   kept in

ward drug cupboard   In patient's locker

3. List community services received:

   1. *Receives none*

   2.

   3.

4. List information received from the community/other hospitals

No letter from the GP.

<u>Outline of planned medical care</u>

Hamilton - Russell traction — 5lb weight
Theatre Monday, July 14, 1976, for crossed
Garden screws.

<u>Summary of main points in nursing history</u>

In view of the inferences made from the
nursing history and the planned medical
care, the following are identified as
problems requiring nursing intervention.

1. *Pain in (R) leg*
2. *Incontinence*
3. *Deafness*
4. *Anxiety over facial hair*
5. *Pressure areas*
6. *Skin damage (R) leg*
7. *Sudden dependency for daily living activities*
8. *Risk of physical postoperative complications.*
9. *Patient will be alone all day following discharge*
10. *Patient's bedroom is upstairs and toilet is downstairs.*
11. *Daughter has disc trouble.*
12. *Ensuring continuity of care and continued progress on discharge*

Care plan for Mrs Doris Adams

Date identified	Problem	Type	Goal	Date begun	Nursing action	Discontinued	Outcome/ Evaluation
9/6	Pain in R. leg	A	Minimise pain	9/6	Refer to history for previous coping mechanisms	9/6	
				9/6	Administer Distalgesic tabs. as prescribed		
				9/6	Explain traction will reduce pain in leg	9/6	
				9/6	Apply Hamilton-Russell traction with 5 lb weight	14/6	Patient says pain is minimal.
				9/6	Use 2 nurses when turning patient		Patient's facial expression is less tense and no tachycardia present
				13/6	Explain pre- and post-operative procedures so as to prepare patient psychologically for surgery.		
				13/6	Give nitrazepam (Mogadon) 10.00 pm as prescribed.	13/6	
				14/6	Administer papaveretum (Omnopon) post-operatively as prescribed and record effect.		
				14/6	Support R. leg on pillow when in left lateral position to prevent pull on wound	14/6	
				14/6	Allow daughter to visit same day as operation	14/6	
9/6	Incontinence	A	Promote continence	9/6	Eliminate cause due to time lapse from falling to being admitted to ward	9/6	Patient had a bedpan in casualty
				9/6	Refer to history for details of incontinence	9/6	Intermittent burning on micturition for the last 3 months. Has had no treatment
				9/6	Refer to history for previous coping mechanisms	9/6	Daughter unaware of the problem as patient does all the washing
				9/6	Perform and chart ward urinalysis	9/6	NAD
				9/6	Perform rectal examination to eliminate faecal impaction as a contributary cause	9/6	Rectum was empty
				9/6	Ensure a minimum of 2 litres/day fluid intake 200 ml 2-hrly between 8.00am and 10.00 pm and 100 mL 2-hrly between 12 mn and 6.00am daily	9/6	Check target is being reached by reference to fluid balance chart
				9/6	Record intake and output chart indicating whether patient is continent.		

Care plan for Mrs Doris Adams

Date identified	Problem	Type	Goal	Date begun	Nursing action	Discontinued	Outcome/ Evaluation
				9/6	Offer bedpan 2-hrly and when requested	15/6	
				10/6	Obtain MSU for culture and sensitivity	10/6	Result showed coliforms 100,000 organisms
				12/6	Explain reason of incontinence to patient		
				15/6	Offer commode 2-hrly and when requested		
				15/6	Ask the patient to stop and restart the flow of urine to make the patient conscious of a means of control		
				20/6	Administer co-trimoxazole (septrin) tab. 10.00am–10.00pm as prescribed.	25/6	Patient was continent day and night when discharged home
9/6	Deafness	A	Use normal coping mechanism	9/6	Refer to history for previous coping mechanisms	9/6	Patient has a private post-aural and an NHS aid Patient is poor at lip-reading
				9/6	Inform all staff of patient's deafness	9/6	
			Participate in 2-way communication	9/6	Speak slowly, in deep tone, facing the patient		
				9/6	Check daily that aid is working	9/6	Aid not working due to corroded battery
				9/6	Ensure aid is always within reach of the patient		
				14/6	Allow patient to wear aid until anaesthetised	14/6	
9/6	1. NHS aid not working	A	Restore aid to working condition	9/6	Send cadet to the Hearing aid centre and wait for aid to be repaired	9/6	Aid in working condition again
9/6	2. Patient, daughter and some staff unaware of the routine care of a hearing aid	A	Perform routine check on aid and know procedure if aid requires attention	9/6	Obtain Hearing Aid Centres booklet on general maintenance of aid	9/6	
				9/6	Inform all nurses where to send aid to be repaired		
				11/6	Explain general care of aid to patient and daughter with reference to booklet at 7.00pm	11/6	
				12/6	Supervise patient is checking aid daily		On discharge the patient with help from daughter was able to check her own hearing aid
				12/6	Arrange teach-in for staff on the maintenance of a hearing aid	14/6	Staff can demonstrate maintenance of a hearing aid

Care plan for Mrs   Doris Adams

Date identified	Problem	Type	Goal	Date begun	Nursing action	Discontinued	Outcome/ Evaluation
9/6	Anxiety over facial hair	A	Continue usual coping mechanism	9/6	Refer to history to establish usual coping mechanisms	9/6	
			Maintain dignity	9/6	Ask daughter to bring battery razor	9/6	
				9/6	Draw screens before using razor		Patient eventually felt able to approach the nurses to help her to use her razor
				9/6	Consider patients embarrassment at having to share her coping mechanism		
9/6	Pressure areas	P	Prevent pressure sores	9/6	Turn patient and chart change of position 2-hrly		
				9/6	Explain reason for turning so as to obtain patients co-operation		
				9/6	Encourage use of poly-perch and bed sides to ease own position		
				9/6	Place pillow under R. calf to prevent pressure on heel from traction	14/6	
				9/6	Check traction spreader remains clear of foot daily	14/6	Pressure areas remained intact
				9/6	Record any deterioration in pressure areas		
				9/6	Keep pressure areas dry		
				9/6	Re-apply traction bandages to R. leg daily	14/6	
				9/6	Observe and report any signs of allergy, skin damage, circulatory impairment	14/6	Toes remained warm and pink
				9/6	Ask patient daily if skin itches under the Elastoplast extensions	14/6	No sign of skin damage or allergy from the traction when completely removed on 14/6/76
9/6	Sudden dependency for daily living activities	A	Retain some control over daily living activities. To maintain maximum independence as condition and treatment will allow				
	(a) Nutrition		Maintain adequate nutrition.	9/6	Organise turn rota, so patient is sitting upright at mealtimes	16/6	
				9/6	Allow patient to feed herself		
				9/6	Allow patient to select food from the choice menu		Patient enjoys her food and selects wisely from the choice menu

Care plan for Mrs Doris Adams

Date identified	Problem	Type	Goal	Date begun	Nursing action	Discontinued	Outcome/ Evaluation
				17/6	Sit to table for meals		
(b) Hydration			Maintain adequate hydration	9/6	Give fluids in a feeder so patient is independent even in a lateral position		No difficulty in reaching 2 litres/day target
				9/6	Observe patient's liking for milk and Horlicks. Milk at 11.00am and 3.00 pm. Horlicks at 8.00pm		
(c) Elimination			Maintain one bowel action daily	9/6	Explain the necessity for bedpans until operation is over		
				9/6	Advise patient on need for roughage in diet	16/6	Patient chooses meals containing roughage
				9/6	Give tab. Dulcolax 10.00 pm if no bowel action for 2 days		Patient's normal bowel pattern maintained
				9/6	Record bowel action on temperature chart		
(d) Hygiene			Attend to own personal hygiene before being discharged	9/6	Bedbath encouraging patient to help		
				16/6	Provide facilities for patient to attend to own teeth before breakfast and after supper.		
				21/6	Provide privacy for patient to wash herself while sitting at the sink	24/6	Patient has no difficulty in coping with this activity
(e) Mobility		A	Walk with a frame assisted by 2 people by the 5th postoperative day.	9/6	Arrange patient's day to be free for physiotherapy at 10.15am Mon – Fri		
				9/6	Encourage R-foot flexion and extension when turning patient to stimulate the circulation		
			Walk unaided with frame by the 10th postoperative day	9/6	Explain and encourage the use of polyperch and bed sides to assist mobility in bed.		
				15/6	Ask daughter to bring in a pair of comfortable walking shoes.	15/6	
				15/6	Allow patient to sit in a chair for 2-hr if tolerated but do not allow to weight bear	17/6	
				15/6	Observe for postural hypotension when standing patient and report		Patient experienced no dizziness on standing and no significant change in blood pressure

Care plan for Mrs Doris Adams

Date identified	Problem	Type	Goal	Date begun	Nursing action	Discontinued	Outcome/ Evaluation
				15/6	Support R. leg on stool to avoid dependent oedema and contracture of hip and knee.		
				17/6	Use frame and 2 people to transfer patient from bed to chair		
				19/6	Walk patient with frame and 2 people to table, toilet and bed		
				20/6	Reduce assistance gradually as patient's ability to mobilise increases		Patient was walking with just a frame on the 9th postoperative day, 23.6.76.
9/6	Risk of physical post-operative complications	A	Minimise risk of postoperative complications by: Prepare patient physically preoperatively.				
				12/6	Inform physiotherapist of intended surgery so assessment for chest physiotherapy can be made	12/6	
				12/6	Assist doctor to obtain specimen of blood to investigate Hb, urea and electrolytes	12/6	
				13/6	Make available patient's current chest X-ray; ECG; biochemical results for the anaesthetist	13/6	
				14/6	Give nil orally after light breakfast at 7.00 am	14/6	
				14/6	Perform skin prep to R. leg	14/6	
				14/6	Perform pubic shave		
				14/6	Put theatre gown on; tape to wedding-ring; offer bedpan	14/6	
				14/6	Give premedication as prescribed	14/6	
			Identify potential physical postoperative complications and take action to try to prevent them from becoming actual problems.				

Care plan for Mrs Doris Adams

Date identified	Problem	Type	Goal	Date begun	Nursing action	Discontinued	Outcome/ Evaluation
14/6	Obstruction to airway	P	Maintain clear airway	14/6	Nurse in lateral position on return from theatre with one pillow		Suction was not needed.
				14/6	Have suction available and in working order	14/6	Patients respirations remained regular, without effort and within a range of 16–20/min and she showed no sign of cyanosis
				14/6	Observe patient's respirations and colour, and report any change	14/6	
						14/6	
14/6	Inadequate ventilation	P	Breathe adequately	14/6	Administer oxygen at 4 litres/min. for the first 4 hours postoperatively via a Ventimask		Patient's colour remained good when oxygen was removed at 8.00 pm
				14/6	Introduce more pillows when BP returns to preoperative reading or above	14/6	
						14/6	
14/6	Disturbance of fluid and electrolyte balance	P	Minimise the disturbance to fluid and electrolyte balance	14/6	Maintain infusion as prescribed	15/6	
				14/6	Reapply bandage to infusion splint am and pm, and check for pain; and inflammation		No pain, local oedema or inflammation observed around infusion site
				14/6	Observe and chart amount of drainage into 3 Redivac drains onto the TPR chart	15/6	
				14/6	Observe and record wound leakage, amount and type	16/6	
				14/6	Record hourly pulse and BP until reviewed at 6.00 pm by doctor		
				14/6	Give oral fluids and diet when tolerated	14/6	
				14/6	Record TBR, BP 4-hrly		
				15/6	Assist doctor to obtain specimen of blood for urea and investigation	15/6	

Care plan for Mrs   Doris Adams

Date identified	Problem	Type	Goal	Date begun	Nursing action	Discontinued	Outcome/ Evaluation
14/6	Injury while under anaesthetic	P	Protect patient from injury while under anaesthetic	14/6	Inform theatre of the need for a sheepskin for theatre table to protect pressure areas	14/6	Pressure areas remained in good condition when checked on return to ward
	Injury to top lip	A		14/6	Inform doctor of injury	14/6	
				14/6	Apply Savlon cream to lip prn		
						16/6	Small cut was healed in 2 days
	Infection of wound	P	Prevent wound from becoming infected	14/6	Recharge 3 Redivac drains prn	16/6	
				14/6	Remove Redivac drains when no drainage for 24 hr	16/6	
				14/6	Redress wound 1st day postop. and then only prn, using an aseptic technique		
				14/6	Record condition of wound when redressed		
18/6	Small drainage from wound	A	Establish if infection present and to treat	18/6	Take wound swab for culture and sensitivity		Swab was sterile
				18/6	Cleanse wound with Dakin's solution		
9/6	Patient will be alone all day following discharge	A	Dress/undress without assistance before discharge	18/6	Discuss problem with patient's daughter	18/6	Daughter is to take two weeks' holiday starting on the day of discharge
				18/6	Ask daughter to bring day clothes in		
				19/6	Refer patient to occupational therapy department for assessment		Little disorganised at dressing activity but manages without help
				19/6	Make nursing history available for OT dept.		Was able to prepare tea and a sandwich safely in OT dept
				20/6	Arrange transport for patient to attend OT dept on 21.6.76 and 22.6.76 at 2.00pm		
				22/6	Supervise patient's dressing/undressing only and report progress		
			To negotiate steps safely before discharge	22/6	Give daily practice in afternoon at negotiating steps		Negotiates steps in usual manner ie can lead with left or right foot

Care plan for Mrs Doris Adams

Date identified	Problem	Type	Goal.	Date begun	Nursing action	Discontinued	Outcome/ Evaluation
9/6	Patient's bedroom is upstairs and toilet downstairs. One week's delay in delivery of commode	A / A	Provide toilet facilities in patient's own bedroom	22/6	Ring appliance officer to arrange for patient to borrow a commode	22/6	A commode will take one week to deliver
				23/6	Ring appliance officer to arrange for patient to borrow a bedpan	23/6	Will be delivered to patient's home on Friday am
9/6	Daughter has disc trouble	A	Daughter to assist patient if necessary without injury or stress to herself or her job	21/6	Arrange 3 evening sessions with daughter		
				22/6	Demonstrate how frame should be used		
					Demonstrate how patient can negotiate steps — advise her to follow behind as a safety precaution	22/6	
				23/6	Demonstrate how patient can dress/ undress without assistance	23/6	
				24/6	Give details of discharge date; out patient appointment; district nurse's visit; tablets to take at home; and how to give a bedpan	24/6	
				24/6	Discuss cause of patient's injury	24/6	Patient's son will cut hedge in future
9/6	Ensuring continuity of care and continued progress on discharge	A	District nurse to assess patient at home	23/6	Telephone the appropriate centre to arrange for a district nurse to visit on Monday 28.6 pm	23/6	
				23/6	Complete form with the relevant details for the patient to hand to the district nurse	23/6	
				23/6	Make an out patient appointment and arrange for transport	23/6	Out patient appointment arranged for 1.7 ambulance ordered
				23/6	Inform daughter of discharge 28/6 am	23/6	Daughter to arrange 2 weeks holiday son to collect patient
				23/6	Give daughter dressing pack x 3 for district nurse	23/6	

Care plan for Mrs   Doris Adams

Date identified	Problem	Type	Goal	Date begun	Nursing action	Discontinued	Outcome/ Evaluation
				25/6	Remove skin sutures	25/6	Steristrips × 3 Applied to part of wound where healing not complete
	DISTRICT NURSE'S VISIT						
28/6	Wound not fully healed	A	Renew dressing using aseptic technique	28/6	Utilise hospital dressing pack		
				28/6	Requisition dressing packs	28/6	Dressing was renewed
				28/6	Use patient's Sello-tape to secure dressing	28/6	
				28/6	Arrange to visit again Friday 2.7.76	28/6	
28/6	Rash on elbows	A	Identify and treat cause of rash	28/6	Inquire from patient suspected cause	28/6	Patient suspects detergent in sheets as she noticed it before being discharged
				28/6	Advise daughter to apply calamine lotion daily		
28/6	Hazardous use of slippers	A	Prevent another injury	28/6	Advise patient to wear shoes when walking		Assess if advice taken on next visit
	OUTPATIENT DEPARTMENT						
1/7	Fear of being re-admitted due to generalised rash	A	Identify and treat cause of rash and allay anxiety	1/7	Inform doctor of rash	1/7	Septrin rash diagnosed
				1/7	Explain the cause of the rash to the patient, and re-assure that there is no need to be readmitted		
				1/7	Ask patient to complete the Septrin course as only 2 tablets left		
				1/7	Reassure patient the rash will go a few days after completing the tablets		Patient very relieved to know she did not need to be readmitted - her birthday is in 2 days
				1/7	Ask patient to continue applying Calamine lotion		
1/7	2.5cm gap in wound when Steristrips removed	A	Give wound the opportunity of primary healing	1/7	Reapply Steristrips and redress wound		
				1/7	Give patient some Steristrips for the district nurse	1/7	
				1/7	Telephone the district nurse to give information regarding the rash and wound.	1/7	Out patient sister spoke with district nurse

Care plan for Mrs Doris Adams

Date identified	Problem	Type	Goal	Date begun	Nursing action	Discontinued	Outcome/ Evaluation
1/7	Long-term problems	P	Detect any long-term problems which can occur with crossed garden screws	1/7	Give patient another out patient appointment for 6 week's time		
				1/7	Arrange transport to bring patient to clinic in 6 weeks	14/8	Patient attended clinic

Paediatric Nursing History   Date 24/3/79

Name *Julie Bea*   Pet name —   Reg no. *012345*

Age *13 years*   D.o.B. *22/2/66*   Sex *F*   Religion *R/C*   Baptised *Yes*

Address *14 Coronation Street, Salford*

Parent/Guardian *Mrs Bea*   Tel. no. *None*

Accommodation *4 bedroomed council house*

Siblings *Two, sister aged 5, brother aged 2*

Father's occupation *Factory worker*

Mother's occupation *Housewife*

Medical diagnosis *Hyperglycaemia / Unstable diabetic*

Plan of medical treatment *IV fluids; s/c insulin*

Previous medical history

Obstetric history *Normal 40/40*

Place of birth *Maternity hospital*

Infectious diseases *Chicken pox: jaundice*

Recent contact *None*

Vaccinations *Triple vaccine, rubella, BCG*

Previous hospital experience *10 previous admissions for hyperglycaemia in last two years*

Parents' understanding of illness and reasons for hospitalisation

Why did you bring your child to hospital?
'She felt sick when she came home from school. At teatime she vomited her tea so my husband gave her some extra insulin'

What has the doctor told you of your child's illness?
'Says she might have an infection'

How do you feel about it?
'It's a bit of a nuisance ... It seems to be happening so often.'

Will you be able to visit?
'Yes in the day time, and after I've got the tea'

Child's understanding of illness and reasons for hospitalisation

Why did Mummy bring you to the hospital?

'*I was feeling sick before tea and then I sicked my tea. Mum was worried because Dad gave me some extra insulin. I kept wanting to drink.*'

What do you think caused you to become ill?

'*The doctor said I might have an infection*'

What has the doctor told you?   *The same.*

How do you feel about it?

'*I don't mind being in hospital. I know it will make me better.*'

Comfort and maintenance

Mother

Has the child had any pain/discomfort recently?

(1) Headaches in the morning   (2) cramp at night

What did you do to relieve it?   *(1) Nothing   (2) Rub her feet*

Did it help much?

(2) Yes, it takes it away

Child

Have you had any pain recently?   *No.*

What did you do to relieve it?   —

Did it help much?   —

Rest and sleep

Bedtime   *10.30 pm*   Time awakened   *7.45 am*

Easily disturbed   *Sleeps fitfully - gets very hot and sweaty at night*

Position of going to sleep   *Right side*

Dummy   —   Soft Toy   *Snake*   Night time drink   —

Blanket   —

Bed/cot?   *Bed - mother's bed when father on nights*

Rest period/naps   *Falls asleep watching TV after school.*

Hygiene

When does child usually bathe? *Evening – Sundays*

Will you be here to bathe child? *Not necessary*

When does the child usually clean his teeth? *At night*

Nutrition

Appetite *Always hungry*   No. of meals *3, breakfast, lunch, tea*

Eating utensils *Knife and fork*

Food likes *New potatoes with lots of butter, chips, peas, meat, sausages*

Food dislikes *Cauliflower, cabbage, green beans*

Fluids drunk: water *Yes*   coffee *No*   milk *Yes*   soft drinks *No*

      tea *Yes*   sugar *Saccharin*   squash *Diabetic*

Cup/beaker/bottle *Cup*

Has illness made any difference to eating/drinking habits?
Couldn't eat this evening. Can't stop drinking

Special diet
Controlled carbohydrate intake – 180g daily

Elimination

Bowel habits *1 x daily*   Time of day *6 pm*   Altered by illness *Yes, 0 x today*

How is request made *Toilet*   Potty/Toilet *Toilet*

Frequency of passing urine *Every 15 minutes today*

General questions

Allergies *None*

School attended *Clear View Open Air School for Delicate Children*

Health visitor/school nurse *Mrs Adams*

Has child been away from home before? *Yes*

Where and with whom? *Hospital – 10 previous admissions*

How did he react? *Settles well – no problems afterwards*

Does child make friends easily?
Yes, but doesn't have any friends at home because she doesn't go to the same school as the others.

Hobbies/Interests? TV, Animals - pet dog

Medicines taken at home? Insulin 40 strength. 34 iu. 7·45 am; 14 iu 4·45 pm
* Type not known

Last taken?
5 pm. Julie and mother will not give injections

Physical assessment

Hearing OK   Sight OK   Wears glasses No.

Movement Full movements of all limbs   Coordination Satisfactory

Handedness Left handed

Temperature 37°C   Pulse 100/min   Respirations 18/min
No smell of acetone

Weight 49 kg (just below 90th percentile)

Gain/loss Steady gain over last 18/12   Height 150 cm (midway between
50th and 25th percentile)

Urinalysis Sugar 2% No Ketones

General appearance Skin dry and flushed. Obese girl. Early secondary sexual
characteristics. Breast development, pubic and axillary
hair. Not menstruating yet.

Dentition Permanent dentition — gross dental caries

Vocabulary/language development
Good vocabulary. Local dialect.

Overall impression of child Pleasant girl, not apprehensive. Admits to eating
biscuits and chocolate. Does not fully understand importance of insulin and
duration of action or sites for injection. Very little exercise - special bus to
delicate school — no games at school. No friends at home.

Overall impression of parent(s) Very protective towards daughter. Believes that
diabetes mellitus is a serious illness and that Julie must be very careful.
Will not give injections of insulin.

Summary of child's problems

1. Hyperglycaemia as a result of inadequate carbohydrate metabolism
2. Dehydration
3. Inadequate understanding of diabetes mellitus
4. Reluctance to give own injections

Summary of parent(s) problems

Mother

1. Lack of understanding of diabetes mellitus and its management

Care Plan

Name *Julie Bea*

Problems	Goals	Nursing Actions	Evaluation
1. Hyperglycaemia as result of inadequate carbohydrate metabolism	1. Julie's blood sugar will return to accepted limits. Urine tests will show ½-1% sugar, no ketones.	1a. Administer insulin as prescribed. b. 180g carbohydrate diet to be given as prescribed by Dr and dietician. c. Observe signs of hypoglycaemia. If present inform H.P. immediately.	4 hourly testing of urine for sugar and ketones. Record findings. 4 hourly observation and recording of pulse and respirations.
2. Dehydration	2. Normal hydration will be achieved by the maintenance of intravenous fluids	2.a. Administer IV fluids at prescribed rate –100ml/hr. b. Check infusion site for leakage or oedema. c. Give assistance when using bedpan. d. Oral fluids may be given as required.	Record all fluid intake and output hourly.

Name *Julie Bea*

Problem	Goals	Nursing Care	Evaluation
3. Inadequate understanding of diabetes mellitus	3. Julie will show competence in the management of diet, exercise and insulin requirements by answering correctly questions pertaining to exercise and insulin required in the course of a normal day and by writing of sample diets. She will also relate when the insulin used has its maximum effect and its duration of action.	3a. Discuss type of control Julie is to aim for and how it may be achieved. b. Refer to dietician for guidance re diet. c. Encourage participation in local BDA activities esp. with other adolescents. d. Supervise Julie in testing urine – question findings and her interpretation of same. e. Supervise Julie in administration of insulin and question understanding of its action.	to produce written samples of suitable diet sheets daily 4 hrly Daily
4. Reluctance to give own injections	4. Julie will administer her own injections of insulin using correct technique and all available sites.	4a. Identify reasons for reluctance to give own injections. b. Demonstrate correct technique of giving insulin. c. Demonstrate and use sites which may be used for injections. d. Provide materials and opportunity for Julie to practise handling of equipment	

Name *Julie Bea*

Problem	Goals	Nursing Care	Evaluation
Mrs Bea 1. Lack of understanding of diabetes mellitus and its management.	1. Mrs Bea will show a developing competence in the management of diabetes mellitus. This will be demonstrated by the writing of sample diet sheets and answering correctly questions relating to exercise and insulin requirements. She will also demonstrate a knowledge of when the insulin used has its maximum effect and its duration of action.	1. a. Assess current knowledge. b. Commence plan of teaching. c. Refer Mrs Bea to dietician for supervision and guidance re diet. d. Demonstrate injection technique. e. Provide materials for Mrs Bea to practise manipulation of equipment. f. Enable Mrs Bea to administer injection g. Refer Mrs Bea to medical social worker and BDA	Test knowledge by questioning and writing possible daily menus 27/3/79 Observe Mrs Bea administering injection 28/3/79
		4 e. Enable Julie to give own injection f. Consult with school nurse re continuing supervision.	Observe Julie giving her own injection

4. Giving Nursing Care

The assessment of patients and the identification of their problems for nursing culminate in the preparation of a plan of nursing care. Such plans, however well prepared, cannot achieve their objectives until the planned actions have been implemented by nurses in the care of their patients.

Systematic Care-Giving

The nursing process has been described as a logical and systematic way of giving patient care. However, to many readers this may sound like meaningless jargon. What, then, is a systematic way of giving care? Broadly speaking, it means that when we plan or give nursing care, we take into account all the factors that might affect patients and the care that they may receive. Much has been said in previous chapters relating to assessment and identification of patient's problems; although these factors play a major role in planning the care a patient should receive, they are not the sole determinants of the actual care given.

When considering the giving of nursing care we must take into account the influence that other factors have on patient care. Nursing does not take place in isolation: it functions within an organisation and environment over which it does not have complete control, and it is frequently dependent on the cooperation of others for the achievement of its goals. For the purpose of discussion here, these factors are described separately, but it should be remembered that in practice they are often difficult to separate because of the influence that one has on another.

Factors Which Influence Nursing Care

Medical diagnosis and doctors' instructions

Nursing and medicine work together in patient care, but each has its own contribution to make. It is usual for nurses to have contact with patients only after patients have presented a problem which they think is amenable to medical intervention. Therefore, the type of nursing care given to a patient is determined to a certain extent by the medical diagnosis. Any nursing care which does not take into account the patient's medical diagnosis is not valid, for such care has ignored the primary problem for which the patient sought help. It is necessary, therefore, to explore ways in which the medical diagnosis, and with it doctors' instructions, influence the type of nursing care given to a patient.

The diabetic patient treated with insulin and dietary control of carbohydrates requires for optimum control of the disease that appropriate sized meals be served at times which coincide with the duration and degree of action of insulin prescribed and administered.

The patient's medical diagnosis and medical treatment therefore determine the nursing actions in meeting the nutritional requirements of the patient. The diagnosis, medical treatment and specific nursing actions in meeting the patient's nutritional requirements also necessitate evaluative nursing actions such as testing the urine of the patient for the presence or absence of glucose and ketones. The presence or absence of these substances in the urine indicates the effectiveness of the nursing and medical actions. These are only two of the ways in which the medical diagnosis of diabetes mellitus and its subsequent medical treatment influence the nursing care a patient receives. The nursing care described is determined by the diagnosis and medical instructions, and not by a wider concept of nursing related to problems amenable to nursing intervention.

Another example of the influence that medical diagnosis and medical instructions have on nursing care is that of the postoperative care of a patient. A patient who has received gastrointestinal surgery may be unable to tolerate oral fluids and diet for a period of time after operation. Even though the patient may complain of hunger or thirst, the nurse may be unable to meet these requirements because of the restrictions placed upon her by the surgeon.

The surgery performed by the surgeon alters the nurse's usual care in meeting the patient's nutritional requirements.

These examples indicate that some of the nursing care a patient receives is dependent upon the medical diagnosis. However, we must bear in mind that nursing has a different contribution to make than medicine to patient care, and therefore the medical diagnosis and doctors' instructions are not the only determinants of nursing care.

Patients' identified problems
The patient's identified problems provide the focal point of nursing care, for it is towards the alleviation of these problems that nursing care is directed. Many nurses are confused by the terminology 'nursing problems', 'patient problems', 'medical problems', and the like, and it is questionable whether problems experienced by patients can be categorised in such a way. It may be preferable to act in terms of problems experienced by patients which may be amenable to care by one or more health care disciplines. Such an example is limited mobility of an elderly person. The doctor may intervene by diagnosing that the patient has osteoarthritis and by prescribing the appropriate medicines and treatment which may maintain or permit greater mobility. The physiotherapist may institute treatment which may maximise what mobility the patient has by the use of heat and exercises. The nurse may assist the patient in the performance of those activities of which he is not capable himself; the nurse assists the patient by arranging the environment in such a way as to permit the elderly person to be as independent as his limited mobility will allow; for example, the patient may be able to feed himself providing that suitable utensils are available. The nurse may also administer the medicines prescribed by the doctor and continue to encourage the patient in performing the exercises commenced by the physiotherapist. In addition, social services may provide help to enable the elderly person to cope with the problems associated with limited mobility.

In such an example, the problem of limited mobility is no more a 'medical problem' than a 'physiotherapy problem', a 'nursing problem' or a 'social problem'. It is a problem experienced by a patient and is amenable in part to care by any of the disciplines mentioned. It is unlikely that action from only one of the disciplines would bring about the desired goals, but working together, this might be achieved.

Patient problems may be divided into two categories:
1. Actual problems
2. Potential problems

Actual problems are problems experienced by the patient at the time the nursing assessment is made. They are readily identifiable in that the patient indicates them or the nurse, using inferential skills, determines their presence and then validates the problem with the patient or others.

An example of such a problem can be found with reference to the care of a baby with cystic fibrosis.

> The nurse, when changing the baby's napkin, notes that the perianal region is red and excoriated. The skin and mucosa of the anus is broken and this is causing obvious discomfort to the baby for he cries when the area is cleansed. The stool passed into the napkin is light brown in colour and of normal amount, consistency and odour. Reference to the baby's feed chart and prescription sheet demonstrates that the baby is taking the required amount of milk feed and in addition is receiving the prescribed amount of supplementary pancreatic enzymes with each feed.
>
> The nurse, using her knowledge of the action of pancreatic enzymes and in particular the sequelae of an imbalance of supplementary pancreatic enzymes and dietary intake, infers in the absence of any other indicators that the cause of the excoriated anus may be that the infant is receiving too much pancreatic enzyme with each feed.

Such a problem is directly amenable to nursing care; the medical staff may be informed of the problem and additional nursing measures instituted with or without being specially instructed to do so by the doctor to promote the healing of the excoriated area and thus alleviate the problem.

Potential problems are not experienced by the patient at the time of assessment but indicators are present that suggest that if no action were taken, problems would arise. For example:

> John, a two-year-old boy, is admitted to hospital complaining of pain in his right knee. His mother states that he has never

been away from home before and that he is a very 'clinging' boy.

The nurse observes that John is very content to sit by his mother's side during the admission interview. He readily answers questions directed to him and he initiates conversation related to the game he is playing. However, when his mother reaches for her handbag, John immediately ceases his game and grasps his mother's skirt. Only after mother assures John that she is not leaving does he return to his game. Further questioning by the nurse reveals that John will not be left with a baby-sitter; if his parents wish to go out he is left with his grandparents.

Acting from her knowledge and observation of interaction between mother and child, the nurse infers that John will almost certainly experience separation anxiety if his mother leaves him in hospital. He has not been separated from his mother before and his behaviour during the interview suggests that he is likely to become very distressed when his mother leaves. Unless some preventative nursing measures are planned and implemented the anxiety suffered may have longer lasting effects after the child returns home. Separation anxiety is therefore a potential problem: John does not display any signs of separation anxiety when his mother is nearby, only when movement suggests that she might leave him.

If the mother can be resident and fully participate in John's care under the supervision of a nurse, then separation anxiety will not become a problem. However, many mothers have other commitments which do not permit them to remain with their child as long as they might like to. In such instances the child might be assigned to the care of a nurse who relates well with the child and who to some extent may act in place of his mother, thus attempting to lessen the degree of separation anxiety which will undoubtedly occur.

Patients' awareness of problems and their willingness
and ability to participate in care
Whether nursing actions achieve their objectives is determined to a large extent by patients' awareness of a problem and their willingness or ability to cooperate with the nurse in reaching the agreed goals of care. Validation of problems and the goals of

care is, whenever possible, of great importance. For only in this way can we work towards gaining cooperation and participation by the patients in their care.

The patient who is unaware of the reason behind the nurse's request that he should not smoke cigarettes on the evening before surgery is unlikely to comply if he is given no indication that to do so might be detrimental to his postoperative recovery. There is no guarantee, having validated that such a problem exists and having provided relevant information, that the patient will comply with the nurse's instructions. The patient must make his own choice as to whether he complies with nursing care. He must be allowed to some extent to decide for himself whether the postoperative risks outweigh the immediate desire to smoke.

However, not all patients are able or capable of taking decisions in relation to their nursing care. The confused, the unconscious and the young are not always able to take such decisions. The cooperation and willingness of others to participate in care is essential whenever a patient remains dependent to any extent for the performance of daily living activities or other activities related to a health problem, for example, the administration of drugs. The elderly patient may require the continuing assistance of relatives, friends or neighbours before the goal of discharge home can be achieved. The young patient is similarly dependent upon others for he is neither legally nor developmentally able to meet his own needs for care.

In such instances, persons other than the patient should be aware of the identified problems and the goals which have been set for his care. The achievement of these goals becomes a shared responsibility between nurse, patient and other carers. There is nothing to be gained from validating a problem with the patient when the patient is an infant. The infant is not capable of caring for himself, therefore it is the infant's mother who is the person who needs to be aware of the problem and of how to cooperate in alleviating the problem.

For example, if a baby has a temporary colostomy to relieve a congenital intestinal obstruction, the mother must feel confident and competent in attending to the stoma before the baby can go home to his family. The district nurse may be able to continue supervision and support of the mother in the care of her baby after discharge but the nurse will not be present to change the baby each time a colostomy action occurs. The nursing care in relation to adjustment to the stoma in this instance should be directed towards the mother. The baby's mother cannot assume full caring responsibilities for her baby until she has been helped to overcome or adjust to her fears and anxieties related to the stoma and until she feels confident and competent in attending to the stoma.

To summarise, nursing care given to patients is influenced by their awareness or perceptions of their problems and their willingness to participate in the care designed to alleviate the problems. In addition, nursing care is also influenced by the dependence of the patient upon others for his continuing care. The degree of dependence as a result of age or handicap necessitates that other carers be aware of the problems and be willing to cooperate in continuing care.

Nurse-doctor relationship
It has been suggested that planned patient care only takes place when an approach such as the nursing process is used. This is not quite true, for planning has previously taken place but usually in relation to the patient's medical diagnosis. Much nursing practice entails the carrying out of doctors' orders and prescriptions, and although this is not the only function of nursing, it is nonetheless a major component. Nursing care has therefore often been seen to be primarily dependent upon medical direction and therefore subservient to medicine. However, despite its appearance of medical dependency, nursing has often been able to influence patient care in many subtle ways. An observation made by Varga demonstrates the influence that nursing and nurses can have on patient care and at the same time illustrates nursing's subservience to medicine.

> Although a nurse may not openly recommend a course of action, she will make it clear in countless subtle ways what she thinks is the proper course of action, but both she and the doctor will preserve the illusion that he always initiates the course of action followed.

The delivery of nursing care determined by a patient's problems requires a very different nurse-doctor relationship than that implied by Varga. It demands an open relationship, one of colleagueship based on mutual trust and acknowledgement of each other's specific contribution to patient care. Only with this type of relationship can we as nurses effectively give care that has been planned to alleviate identified patient problems. This type of relationship does not always exist at present; in order that it might, we must be able to demonstrate why the problems we have identified are problems, and also why the nursing actions we have selected are appropriate.

For many years nurses have been guilty of selecting nursing actions according to personal preference or tradition rather than by making conscious objective decisions about the type of care they will provide. The numerous 'treatments' used to promote the healing of pressure sores is one example of the type of personal preference and traditional nursing actions referred to. Unless we can provide a rationale for our nursing actions, we will find difficulty in discussing with doctors the appropriate course of action to be taken to meet the problems and needs presented by patients. A relationship between nurse and doctor based on mutual trust and understanding of each other's contribution has to be earned and it will not be achieved until we are able to explain what we are doing for patients and why.

Patient care is a joint venture between several health care disciplines, but the ultimate responsibility is normally invested in the doctor. This has considerable implications for nursing care, for the type of nursing care planned for a patient may not always coincide with the treatment planned by the doctor. Take, for example, planning the discharge of a patient. The decision to discharge a patient rests with the doctor and is usually determined by the patient's state of health. However, during assessment, the nurse may have discovered that the mother of a physically handicapped baby is frightened and anxious when participating in the care of the child. She will be expected and encouraged to perform relatively simple exercises with baby at home, but has not yet come to terms with having given birth to a handicapped child. The nurse must discuss with the doctors to determine not only that the child is well enough to be discharged but that the mother feels confident and competent to continue the care of her child at home under the supervision of the community nursing services.

Nursing care planned to help the mother adjust to and cope with a handicapped child may be more difficult to achieve than the medical goal of care for the child and may well take longer. The mother will almost certainly require ongoing support and supervision once she returns home with her child, and it may be advisable for those community nurses who will continue this care to visit the mother and child while in hospital. This cannot be achieved at a moment's notice; it requires collaboration and trust between doctors and nurses.

When doctors and nurses are both engaged in meeting the same identified patient problem, an understanding and acknowledgement of the other's contribution is of particular importance. The example given previously of limited mobility of an elderly person is one such instance when the desired outcome or goal would not be met by the actions of only one of the disciplines mentioned. Each has its own contribution to make and each must acknowledge the other's contribution to patient care. If one discipline fails to acknowledge another's contribution, then goals for care may not be completely achieved and this may give rise to further health problems at a later date.

Resources available

Nursing personnel British nursing is heavily dependent upon learners for the delivery of patient care. This must of necessity influence the type of nursing care given to patients, for those giving the care that has been planned are still acquiring knowledge and expertise in nursing skills. The level of nursing care received by a patient is therefore dependent upon the breadth and depth of knowledge possessed by the nurse and also by her proficiency in performing a range of skills.

Knowledge and skills, although separate entities, are closely linked in the practice of nursing. For example, we may possess a knowledge of asepsis but may not yet have acquired the manual dexterity required for performing an aseptic technique. Conversely, we may be able to manipulate dressing forceps, but without an understanding of the principles underlying asepsis the patient's wound may not be dressed in an aseptic manner.

The links between knowledge and skills are demonstrated in

all aspects of nursing. A nurse may have acquired a high level of skill in interviewing patients and collecting other relevant information, but without a sound underlying knowledge she will find difficulty in identifying patient problems. Likewise, the ability to plan care is dependent upon a knowledge from which to select appropriate nursing actions. The number of choices available to a nurse is determined by her knowledge and previous experience. Evaluation is complicated and requires a good deal of knowledge. Evaluation of nursing care comprises the comparison of the outcome of nursing actions against predetermined goals for care. This is as yet a poorly developed aspect of nursing and requires skill in setting goals and in determining measurable criteria for the achievement of goals.

Not all nurses responsible for caring for patients will have acquired the same level of expertise and knowledge. Consequently, the type of care a patient receives will differ according to the nurse's ability and experience. It would be unrealistic to expect a nurse in the first few months of training to possess and use the same degree of knowledge and skill in her nursing care as the nurse nearing completion of training. These skills have to be learned and developed but not in isolation from each other. The nursing process is a continuous process of assessment, planning, intervention and evaluation. Skills must therefore be learned simultaneously because, as previously discussed, they cannot be separated in practice for they constitute the very actions of nursing: What may differ is the level of competence achieved by nurses in these skills.

Nurse learners at the beginning of training may well be able to administer a structured interview but will need help and guidance in eliciting non-verbal cues given by the patient or relative, if the information given is to be complete. In addition, the patient problems the learners are readily able to identify will be limited to the basic preparation they have received. The nurses will therefore require further help from trained staff to properly assess and identify the patient's problems. Similarly, the choice of nursing actions the nurse learners may select to meet a problem will be limited in the first instance, but with the help of trained staff they will be able to build up a repertoire of nursing actions which they will be able to adapt to meet any given patient problem.

As the nurse learners progress in their training and acquire more knowledge and skills, the number of patient problems they may identify from their assessment will increase and similarly the range of nursing actions they employ in caring will become more varied. In addition, the need for supervision and guidance from trained staff should decrease as the nurses become more experienced so that they assume greater responsibility for the care they are planning and giving to their patients.

To permit nurses in training to fully participate and develop these skills in relation to the knowledge they have gained, wards are required to accommodate a suitable balance of learners at differing stages of training and adequate supervision and guidance from trained staff. Insufficient trained nursing staff and a preponderance of junior student nurses might not permit complete or safe nursing care. The type of nursing care planned and given is therefore dependent upon the resources available, that is, the ability and competence of the nurses giving care.

Equipment   Among the resources to be considered which influence nursing care is the equipment needed to give care. We have to question not only if the equipment required is available but also if it is suitable for the patient.

Whenever we plan care to meet the identified problems of a patient, we run the risk of idealising that care. However much we might strive to reach that ideal, it must be borne in mind that we have to work within the constraints and limits of the organisation in which we are employed.

There are local policies which dictate whether certain items of equipment are allowed to be used and even when they should be used. It might be the policy of the hospital that any patient with a history of epilepsy be nursed with cot-sides on the bed at night. The epilepsy may be well controlled and bear no relation to the patient's current health problems. Nevertheless, the hospital policy may dictate that the nurse, being aware of the patient's previous medical history, include the use of cot-sides in providing a safe environment for the patient. Conversely, the local policy might dictate that certain items of equipment should not be used in giving care. In addition, the hospital's budget may determine the range and number of items of equipment available for use.

When planning care we must therefore consider the availability of equipment we might employ in order to provide that care.

Having ascertained that the required equipment is available, we must also determine whether it is suitable for use by the patient. When undertaking assessment, a nurse may have identified a patient as being at risk from developing pressure sores. The nurse may have considered the use of protective sheepskins but this would be unsuitable if the patient were allergic to wool. Although the equipment might be readily available and previously had been demonstrated to be effective in the prevention of pressure sores, it would be unsuitable for use in this instance: an alternative material or method would have to be used. The absence or availability of equipment and its suitability for use therefore influences the nursing actions selected by a nurse in giving patient care.

Environment
The ward environment or ward design is a very important factor which influences nursing care. There are several types of ward design to be found in our hospitals and each may have a different effect on the type of care a patient might receive. Any one ward design may be both advantageous and disadvantageous for the patient. It is possible that some features of a ward may be the cause of patient problems, while other features may act as a source of strength. For example, a patient nursed in a large Nightingale ward may find difficulty in sleeping at night because of the general noise and disturbance, and yet find the companionship and camaraderie of the other patients a great source of help. Conversely, patients nursed in single rooms may have the privacy they desire but may suffer considerable anxiety because they feel that they cannot readily attract the attention of a nurse. In each of these examples the environment provides a source of strength and yet at the same time gives rise to patient problems. Ward design therefore influences problems experienced by patients and consequently the nursing care that patients receive.

Ward organisation
There are two broad categories of ways in which nurses may be deployed in patient care: task allocation and patient allocation. However, in practice, the division is not as clear cut. To emphasise

how methods of staff deployment influence patient care, let us look at them separately.

Task allocation   This type of staff deployment entails the allocation of tasks or procedures to nurses of differing levels of training and experience. Nurses at the beginning of training are allocated what has been termed 'basic nursing' tasks which include activities such as bedmaking, bathing, the giving of bedpans and urinals. These tasks fall into the category of meeting the needs of patients in activities of daily living. As the nurse learners become proficient in these basic nursing tasks or skills and progress in their training, they take on more technical tasks. Technical nursing tasks are understood to be tasks or procedures such as the changing of surgical dressings, the administration of drugs, the care of intra-venous infusions.

Task allocation results in fragmentation of care. Several nurses may administer nursing care to any given patient and yet no one particular nurse is accountable for that patient's care. With this type of deployment nurses are accountable only for the undertaking and completion of tasks assigned to them; consequently, difficulty may be experienced in focussing on the total needs of the patient. In addition, any communication concerning patient care tends to be one way; from the nurse in charge by way of instructions to the nurses giving care. There is little opportunity for or expectations of the nurses giving care to comment on the patient's response to the nursing care given.

Patient allocation   The other broad category of deployment entails the allocation of nurses to the care of groups of patients in an attempt to lessen the fragmentation of care inherent in task allocation.

The focus of nursing care is the patient and his problems, rather than the tasks to be performed. Within this category are two types of deployment pattern: team nursing and patient assignment.

Team nursing emerged as a means by which more integrated and individualised care might be provided for patients. Instead of all the nurses caring in part for all the patients on a ward, the work-load is divided between teams of nurses each headed by a staff nurse or senior student nurse. The team leader is accountable for planning the care of patients to whom the team is assigned, but remains responsible to the ward sister who acts in a supervisory capacity.

The method of organising patient care employed by the team leader is dependent upon the policy of the ward. While team nursing lends itself well to patient allocation, it is also possible for task assignment to operate in conjunction with it. However, it is generally assumed that team nursing is analogous to patient allocation. For this style of deployment to function effectively, each team must be composed of a balanced mix of nurse learners. Care must be taken in the assignment of nurses to the care of patients to ensure that the nurses are capable of providing the care required of them. It is not sufficient to assume that less ill or dependent patients may be cared for by junior nurses. The plan of care for such patients might include preparation for discharge for which teaching skills are imperative and which will not, as yet, have been acquired by the junior nurse learner.

Each nurse is held accountable for the care she has given or omitted to give at the ward report or patient conference meeting. The reporting by nurses of the care they have given permits two-way communication between the care giver and the ward sister. Decentralisation or delegation of authority to nurses for patient care is essential, but the ward sister, in retaining the over-all responsibility for patient care, remains in a position to supervise, guide and counsel nurse learners in the care they are giving.

Patient assignment involves the allocation of a nurse to the care of a patient or small group of four to five patients. The nurse is then responsible for carrying out the plans of care for those patients throughout a span of duty. Assignment of patients to particular nurses can be done on a day-to-day shift basis, a weekly basis, or ideally for the length of a patient's stay in hospital. Patient assignment does not necessarily mean that nurses will be responsible for assessing their patients' problems and requirements for nursing care, although it does provide an opportunity for them to do so under the guidance and supervision of trained nursing staff. Because the nurse is accountable for only a small number of patients, she is in a better position to recognise and meet the needs of her patients more readily, and fragmentation of care is therefore limited only to changes of shift. However, as with team nursing, whenever patient assignment is practised there is great need to closely match the needs of patients with the levels of skill and knowledge possessed by the nurses who are to care for those patients.

There are benefits which accrue to both patients and nurses when using this style of patient care. Nurses are provided with an opportunity to recognise and meet the total needs of their patients; they are accountable for the nursing care which they provide; and, in addition, they may begin to develop an ability to plan and organise their work according to the priority of care demanded by their patients.

Primary nursing is a concept of deployment new to nursing in British hospitals, but deserves mention in this discussion of patient assignment. It is really an extension of patient assignment: the nurse assigned to a group of patients is totally responsible for their twenty-four hour care until discharge. Primary nursing differs from what is generally understood as patient assignment in that the nurse assigned to the care of a group of patients is a qualified nurse and therefore able to assume total responsibility for the care she plans and gives.

Adaptation of Plans to Practice

The nursing care plan provides a *basis* for action. It should not be seen as a set of instructions to be adhered to rigidly, but rather as a plan of action designed to meet the problems of patients at the time when the plan was made. However, patient problems do not remain static and the other factors, described earlier in this chapter, which influence patient care, rarely remain constant. When giving patient care nurses must of necessity constantly re-assess patient problems, evaluate the care they have given, reorder priorities of care according to the demands of the patient or the needs of others, and in doing so make changes within the broad remit of the care plan.

Changes in Patient Problems

Patient problems are dynamic not static in nature; thus the nursing care required must be constantly updated to keep pace with the patient's changing status. In the first instance the nursing care plan is derived from the initial assessment of the patient: the patient's problems at that time are subject to change and consequently the care also changes. It is during the giving of care that reassessment of problems and nursing care occurs.

While covering the care required to meet the majority of actual and potential patient problems, the nursing care plan cannot possibly anticipate every eventuality that might arise; to do so would make the care plan unmanageable and detract from its value. An illustration of this can be seen in the following example.

> Mr Brown, aged 56 years, has undergone major surgery for the repair of a perforated duodenal ulcer. Among the postoperative problems experienced by Mr Brown is that of pain which may be relieved by the regular administration of prescribed analgesics. Potential problems which may arise as a consequence of surgery and the degree of pain experienced and for which nursing intervention should be instigated are pulmonary congestion and venous thrombosis.

The nursing actions employed in preventing these potential problems from becoming actual problems should rightly be found in the nursing care plan. However, it would be inappropriate for anticipatory nursing actions to be detailed in readiness for the event of these potential problems becoming actual problems. This may be done if and when the change from potential to actual problems occurs. The change in nursing care results from evaluation of the care given previously. The nursing care plan is therefore adapted to meet the changed problems of the patient.

The example shows the way in which the care plan is adapted when potential problems progress to become actual problems. Conversely, evaluation of care and reassessment of patients' problems while giving care may reveal that previously identified problems are no longer present. If this were so, then to proceed with the care as planned would also be inappropriate. For example, a patient has a problem of raised body temperature (40°C) caused by a bacterial infection. The nursing care planned to alleviate this problem might include the use of an electric fan to cool the environment, in addition to the administration of antibiotics and antipyretic agents prescribed by the doctor. The nurse, in evaluating the effectiveness of the nursing care given, notes that the patient is no longer flushed, neither does he complain of fever. These subjective observations are confirmed by the nurse when, after taking the patient's oral temperature, the clinical thermometer reads 36.5°C. The problem of pyrexia has been alleviated.

To continue the nursing care planned would be inappropriate, for cooling the environment when the patient has a normal body temperature might result in further discomfort for the patient. The nursing care plan has to be adapted to take into account the changed status of the problem. The immediate problem of pyrexia no longer exists, but because the bacterial infection causing the pyrexia has not yet been eliminated, it becomes a potential problem. This potential problem requires continuing monitoring and the administration of treatments prescribed by the doctor.

Another way in which the status of patient problems might result in the adaptation of the nursing care plan is the presence of new and perhaps unexpected problems in the course of giving care. The initial assessment, as we now know, may not reveal all the problems that a patient might experience. The progress of the patient's illness or recovery may give light to problems at differing times during his stay in hospital. No matter how comprehensive the initial nursing history, the information gathered is dependent upon that given voluntarily by the patient or other carer. The patient or his carer may not at that time feel ready to divulge specific fears or anxieties pertaining to the hospital admission. Such information may be offered at a later date once the relationship with the nurse has been more fully established. Assessment of patient problems is not a once only event, it must continue throughout the patient's time in hospital in conjunction with giving care and evaluating the care given. Only in this way can the care given be appropriate to the problems experienced by patients at any given time.

The examples given so far demonstrate that the nursing care required by patients alters from that previously planned when new problems are identified or the nature of the problem changes or when both occur. The nurse providing the immediate care will be aware of the change in the patient's problems and will alter her nursing care accordingly. However, the care plan which is available to other nurses and health workers will not be appropriate for his problems at that time. Whenever reassessment of patient problems or evaluation of care given results in a change in the type of nursing care required, an entry must be made to that effect on the nursing care plan. It may be sufficient to enter on the care plan when a problem and its subsequent nursing care ceased, but when a problem changes in status from potential to actual or vice versa, additional instruction for nursing care will be required. The same is required with the identification of new patient problems. It may be helpful at this point to refer back to the chapter on planning patient care; for in adapting plans to practice one is 'updating' the care plan. Patient problems are dynamic in nature and the nursing care plan must also be dynamic.

Changes in Priorities for Nursing Care

Just as patient problems change in the course of time, so also do priorities for care. The ordering of priorities is determined not only by an individual patient's problems but by the demands made on the nurse by other patients and health care staff.

In the first instance, the extent and urgency of the patient's problems dictate the priority of action accorded to them; for example, an unconscious patient's first priority will be the maintenance of a clear airway, nutrition and elimination. These are basic physiological functions which must be met in order to sustain life. Other problems of the patient are accorded lower priority, but as the patient regains consciousness and is able to maintain his own basic physiological functions, social interaction and rehabilitative nursing actions will assume greater priority. Alterations in the patient's condition, and therefore in the priority of care required, must be constantly reassessed.

However, except in special settings, for example, intensive care units, nurses are rarely responsible for the care of only one patient; it is usual for nurses to care for a small group of patients. Therefore, the demands for care made by a group of patients on the nurse will also determine the priority of care given to each. The heavy demands made by one patient may mean that the care for another has to be reassessed. A decision may have to be made as to what nursing care might safely be delegated to others, or perhaps left to another time. At times when demands made on nursing staff outnumber the nurses available, nursing care that has been planned may, of necessity, be undertaken by another. Is the patient capable of undertaking a particular item of care himself, or perhaps his relative? Whenever others are involved in the care of a patient, it may be necessary to change the ordering of the care planned. If it is known that a relative will be visiting at a specific time it may be possible to defer certain items of care so that they might participate. However, we must consider whether the nursing care deferred is appropriate for another to perform. Although a young man might well be able to wash his mother, it might not be appropriate for him to do so. He might, however, assist her in walking to the bathroom or getting out of bed and sitting in a chair.

Other health care disciplines also participate in patient care, therefore nursing care that has been planned for any particular patient must also fit in with that offered by others. A request from the X-ray department for a patient to attend for examination may require a change in the nursing care plan, a reordering of care or special preparation. If the physiotherapist is delayed it may be necessary to defer the administration of specifically pres-cribed drugs until such time as the physiotherapist can be present, for example, inhaled mucolytics prior to chest physiotherapy.

Changes in Resources Available

Resources in the form of nursing personnel to care for the patients are not always stable. Reference has been made earlier to the reliance on nurse learners in British nursing for the provision of patient care. Although every effort may be taken to match the patients' needs for care with the skills and knowledge of the nurses caring for them, this is not always practical. Whenever such a position arises it may be necessary to adapt the care given to the level of expertise of the nurse. Alternatively, the care planned may be given by or under the supervision of trained nurses, but this may require reordering of care and priorities. Likewise, the availability or non-availability of equipment needed in providing nursing care may require adaptation of the nursing care plan.

The nursing care plan provides a written communication of the care a patient requires. However, we have seen the ways in which extraneous factors influence how and if the care planned is administered. The nursing care plan is essential as a guide to the care required, but changes in problems, priorities and resources necessitate adaptation of the plans in practice. To adhere rigidly to the plan of action without considering the dynamics of patient and nursing care, would detract from its value. As changes occur, so also must nursing care and with it the plan of care.

Handing Over Patient Care Using Nursing Care Plans

The nursing care plan has so far been discussed in terms of its compilation and adaptation to the immediate future needs of the patient. What has not been discussed is the use of the nursing care plan as a means of communicating the nursing care required by any one patient to those nurses involved in his care. The nursing care plan is itself a written communication of a patient's nursing requirements and in addition it may serve as a basis for verbal communication when handing over care at change of shifts.

The Nursing Care Plan as a Written Means of Communication

Let us consider the first function of the nursing care plan, that of providing a written form of communication. No matter what type of staff deployment is used, several nurses may be involved in the care of a patient during the course of a day and this number may be further increased depending on the patient's length of stay in hospital. Sickness, days off-duty and internal rotation of night duty all contribute to the necessity for several nurses to be involved in the care of any one patient. The delivery of care by a number of nurses necessitates accurate communication of a patient's needs for care and his response to the nursing care given. Accurate communication is essential for nursing care to be effective and also for the effects of fragmentation of care to be lessened. The nursing care plan has the potential for providing such accurate means of communication.

In writing out the patient's problems, the nursing goal and the nursing care required to meet these goals, any nurse caring for that patient has a written source of reference to which to refer. This is of particular importance when one nurse is assigned to the care of several patients. It might not be appropriate or safe for the nurse to attempt to memorise every detail of care required. However, if a written nursing care plan is available and accessible for reference, continuity of care and safe care may be more readily assured.

There are times when the nursing care plan may be the only source of communication available, for example, if a nurse falls sick or an emergency in the ward necessitates that another takes over a patient's care. The nursing care plan should therefore contain sufficient concise information to permit it to be the only form of communication. It should contain a statement of the current problem(s), goal(s), nursing actions selected to meet the problem(s) and a time or date when evaluation of care given should be made. If the nursing care plan is to act as an efficient means of written communication it must be revised as the patient's nursing care changes to meet his present needs. A patient's nursing care on returning to the ward following surgery may differ considerably from that which was required preoperatively. There may be instructions from the surgeon to be followed, for example, analgesia, positioning of body or limbs and specific observations to be made. In addition, the patient's degree of dependence on the nurse may have increased. For a period of time the patient may be unable to meet his own needs in daily living activities, he may require assistance from the nurse. Unless the nursing care plan is altered to this effect the plan will not provide an effective up-to-date means of communication.

The Nursing Care Plan as a Basis for Verbal Communication

It is usual practice when patient care is handed over from one nurse to another that a verbal report is given, one to the other. The nursing care plan may complement the verbal report which takes place at change of shifts. It may act as a basis or framework from which to communicate the patient's nursing care to others.

The use of the nursing care plan which includes patient's identified problems and the goals for care, focusses the report on those aspects of care which are nursing. Various authors have commented that usually delegated medical care is reported upon the expense of nursing information. For example, at change of shift a nurse may be informed when a patient last received analgesia, or the present rate of an intravenous infusion but less frequently the patient's response to treatment, his preferences or what he is able to do for himself. The performance of delegated medical care is an important part of nursing care but it is not the only component of nursing. The use of the nursing care plan helps to ensure that verbal reports contain such information that will help the nurse to care effectively for her patients.

The nursing care plan may therefore act as a means of communicating patient care in two ways: in its written form and as a framework for verbal reporting. These methods of communication may be employed between individual nurses caring for a patient or at 'ward report', at which time the efficacy of nursing care planned for particular patients may be discussed.

Nurse-to-Nurse Communication of Nursing Care

Communication between individual nurses caring for a patient, may take place at the patient's bed side. Patients who are able may be encouraged to participate in their care and in particular in that care planned for the immediate future. Patient participation at this juncture provides an opportunity for nurses both to validate the presence of problems and to discuss with the patient how the problem(s) might be alleviated. In this way differing expectations by nurse and patient in respect of care given and received may be narrowed and realistic goals can then be set and achieved.

The Patient-care Planning Conference

The patient-care planning conference is a time at which skills of problem identification, the setting of goals, selection of nursing actions and use of evaluative measures may be developed and practiced.

We know that nurses at different stages of training possess different levels of knowledge and skill. The opportunity to contribute to and question the rationale behind identified patient problems and suggested nursing care is an invaluable aid to active learning by the nurse learner and ultimately to patient care.

The identification of patient problems and the selection of appropriate nursing actions are skills which have to be learned and practised if nurse learners are to become safe practitioners. These skills may be acquired by 'trial and error' learning but this method of learning is time-consuming and, more seriously, may cause the patient unnecessarily long periods of dependency or perhaps even harm. For example, patients at risk from developing pressure sores may go unrecognised until reddened areas appear, or the application of spirit to the patient's heels as a method of preventing sores may result in cracking of the skin and subsequent sores.

The patient-care planning conference provides an outlet for the collective knowledge and skills of the ward staff. The identified problems of a patient and the nursing care planned for that patient may be brought to the conference for discussion. For example, a nurse learner recently assigned to an orthopaedic ward may be unfamiliar with problems experienced by patients on skeletal traction and with specific nursing methods employed in the care of such patients. The nurse learner's previous experience and knowledge may enable her to identify common problems and she might also receive help and guidance in this respect from another more senior or trained nurse. However, the nurse learner's assessment of the patient's experienced difficulties and problems is ultimately dependent upon the extent of her knowledge and experience. The nurse learner may have correctly identified that the patient has problems associated with mobility but might not possess the particular knowledge and skills required to help the patient cope with this problem. However, discussion at the patient-care planning conference of alternative methods of lifting and turning patients will ensure that the most appropriate method is selected to meet this particular patient's problem.

In providing the nurse learner with an opportunity to present to other members of the ward staff the findings of her assessment and the subsequent plan of care, the learner is enabled to extend her knowledge and enlarge her scope for nursing care. Moreover, the nurse learner is encouraged to develop a critical approach to the selection of the most appropriate nursing actions through being exposed to suggestions for alternative methods of care.

Advantages and Disadvantages of Using the Nursing Process

The use of a systematic approach to nursing care, that is, the nursing process, has received many accolades and criticisms from experienced nurses. Perhaps it has become evident from the text what these accolades and criticisms might be. However, the advantages to be gained and the possible disadvantages in using the nursing process should be made explicit if the reader is to judge the benefits or otherwise which might accrue from its use in the practice of nursing.

Criticisms and Disadvantages

The most common criticisms made are those of the length of time required to make a nursing assessment and plan care and the need for more nurses. These two criticisms are really one; they relate to lack of time or shortage of nurses. How long does it take to make a nursing assessment and plan nursing care for a patient? It is not possible to give a precise answer to that question for it will depend on the extent and depth of the assessment, the number of patient problems identified and the amount of individual nursing care required by the patient. The length of time required is also dependent upon the experience of the nurse making the initial assessment and plan of care. Undoubtedly, at first the nursing assessment is lengthy, but as the nurse becomes experienced and skilled, the time taken is considerably less. This is no different from the learning of any other skill. When a nurse removes sutures from a wound for the first time she is very slow and unsure, but as she gains experience in handling the instruments and materials the procedure is not only performed more skilfully but also takes much less time.

The efficacy of subjecting a sick patient to a battery of questions is another criticism closely related to that of the length of time necessary to make a nursing assessment. In reply to this criticism, firstly I would hope that no patient is subjected to a battery of questions. A properly conducted interview is a two-way process of exchange of information, not an interrogation which the criticism implies. What ought to be considered is the time at which the initial assessment should take place. If a patient enters hospital as an arranged admission it would seem most appropriate for the information required to be obtained shortly after the patient's arrival on the ward. A nursing assessment made at that time would rapidly become part of the ward 'admission procedure'.

However the criticism usually relates to the patient who is admitted to hospital acutely ill. Is it ethical to interview a patient who is suffering considerable pain, is dyspnoeic or confused? Such criticism demonstrates a lack of understanding of the meaning of assessment. The nursing assessment does not solely consist of taking a nursing history; it also involves observational skills and the seeking of information from other sources (see chapter 2, Assessment of Patient Problems). When a patient is admitted to a ward, the nurse assigned to the care of that patient will already be in possession of some information relating to the patient. It is usual practice when a patient is admitted to hospital via the Accident and Emergency Department for the admitting doctor to inform the ward of the patient's name, provisional diagnosis, general condition and any specific medical treatment required on admission to the ward. This advance information used in conjunction with the nurse's own observations of the patient on arrival to the ward enables the nurse to determine whether a more thorough assessment should be made at this time. I emphasise 'a more thorough assessment' because a preliminary nursing assessment has been made. It may be that the outcome of this preliminary assessment would be to defer the more formal nursing assessment until later. However, much information relating to the patient might be gained from the person(s) accompanying the patient which might be of use in planning that patient's nursing care after the immediate emergency care has been instituted.

The patient, when more comfortable or lucid, may provide or confirm personal information given at a later date. While it is appropriate that the initial assessment should be made at or shortly after the patient's admission to the ward, there are times when this is not possible. At such times the use of other sources, for example, relatives and previous medical and nursing notes, assumes greater significance in providing information on which to plan care for the immediate future. Moreover, it is important to stress that the initial nursing assessment only provides the foundation for further assessments made during the course of nursing care.

Another criticism made of the nursing process is the degree of responsibility apportioned to nurse learners in requiring them to identify patient problems and to plan and evaluate care accordingly. Undoubtedly, this criticism requires careful consideration. An easy answer would be that nurse learners are at present required to provide nursing care with sometimes little guidance. However, such nurse learners may be unaware of the rationale behind their actions, only that they have been told to perform some aspect of nursing care by a more senior nurse or have observed others doing so. Nursing care performed using a problem-solving approach demands more of the nurse learner: care is much less likely to be mere routine.

In identifying patient problems, nurse learners know to what aims their nursing actions are directed and must therefore become aware of why they have selected the nursing actions used. This is indeed very much more demanding of the nurse learners: instead of simply performing care as directed, the nurse learners are required to account for the care they are giving. Can this truly be considered a criticism or disadvantage of using the nursing process? It can, but only if the nurse learner is left unsupervised and unguided. Nurse learners cannot be held totally responsible for the identification of patient problems and the planning and evaluation of nursing care; this responsibility must remain with a senior or trained nurse. As the nurse learners become more experienced and knowledgeable they will undoubtedly feel more ready to take on more responsibility for assessing patient problems and planning nursing care.

The amount of responsibility for patient care delegated to nurse learners should be dependent upon their ability and previous experience. The use of the nursing process does not remove patient responsibility from the trained nurses: the trained nurses retain this responsibility and this is demonstrated by their supervision and guidance of the nurse learner when identifying patient problems and planning care. They also retain responsibility for ensuring that the care planned is given and that its effectiveness is evaluated.

Advantages

The advantages of using the nursing process in patient care may be broadly divided into two categories: those pertaining to the patient and those pertaining to the nurse caring for the patient. Let us first consider those advantages which accrue to the patient.

Advantages for the patient

Reference is made in chapter 2 to the relationship built up between patient and nurse when a nursing history is taken. Experience demonstrates that this relationship with one nurse is of great importance to patients. Patients have reported that the interest demonstrated by the nurse in gaining the type of information requested and the time spent on this at the beginning of their hospital experience, made them feel that they were individuals and not 'just another patient'. They were able to identify a particular nurse with whom they could relate and with whom they felt more ready to share their happinesses and their worries and anxieties.

The importance of this relationship for patients cannot be overemphasised. It has been our experience that many nurses, both trained and learners, are at first hesitant to ask the patient about some of the areas outlined in chapter 2. These nurses expressed concern that such lines of enquiry might cause embarrassment or resentment or both in the patient. Closer examination of their feelings by these nurses usually reveals that it is they who feel embarrassment rather than their patients to whom they direct this concern. This gives rise to the need to help nurses to develop interviewing and counselling skills in order that they might conduct interviews without causing embarrassment or resentment in their patients.

In addition to the relationship formed between patient and nurse, the assessment of a patient's problems when he is first admitted to hospital encourages his active involvement and participation in care. Whenever possible, the patient becomes an active participant in his care rather than a passive receiver of care. Moreover, if patients contribute to the identification of their own problems and needs, it is very much more likely that the goals of both patient and nurse will be congruent. For example, a patient who understands the need for an uncomfortable nursing task such as changing position two to four hourly, or a seemingly irrelevant request to drink 3 litres of fluid a day, is very much more likely to comply with the plan of nursing care and therefore the goals for care are more likely to be met.

Apart from understanding the need for nursing care, the use of the nursing process and in particular the concept of patient participation underlying it, permits the patient greater control over what nursing care is planned. There is much controversy as to where the nursing care plan should be kept: should it be kept in a central office or nursing station or should it be kept at the patient's bedside. If the patient has contributed to the identification of his own problems for care there would seem to be no worthwhile reason against the nursing care plan being kept at the bedside. The patient might then be able to refer to it himself. Such access to the nursing care plan provides the patient with an opportunity to question care. The patient is therefore able to retain some degree of independence in the control of his life while in hospital.

Advantages for Nurses Caring for Patients
The relationship which is formed between patient and nurse when the nursing assessment is made is also advantageous for the nurse. During this interchange of information the nurse gains a better understanding of the patient as a person. She is thus better equipped to plan his nursing care and assess his response to that care. The nursing care planned as a consequence of identified patient problems becomes focussed on the patient rather than on the disease from which he suffers. Of course medical delegated care arising from the patient's medical diagnosis will still play a major part of the nursing care provided but in addition, the nurse will be able to identify her own contribution to patient care.

But what of the practical advantages for the nurse in using the nursing process? The advantages are best discussed in terms of the benefits which accrue to individual nurses caring for groups of patients and those which accrue to the nurse in charge of a ward. The nurse learners who are able to participate in the planning of patient care as well as its implementation are likely to reach a better understanding of the rationale behind those nursing actions. Instead of simply being instructed to perform the care required for a patient, they actively assist in the planning of care. This active learning in the practice of nursing is more readily linked with the more formal ongoing nursing education.

The nursing care plan itself provides security for the nurse for she has a written plan of action to refer to. This plan details not only the patient's problems and the appropriate nursing care required but also a statement of the goals for each of these actions. The nurse is aware of what she intends to achieve with the patient: she is also therefore in a position to determine the effectiveness of her nursing care.

Being accountable for the nursing care she has given permits the nurse to reflect on what she has achieved during the course of a shift or over a period of several days. This sense of achievement gained from identifying patient problems, planning and implementing care and evaluating care against goals set is considerably rewarding to the nurse. She is able to take a personal interest in both the progress of her patients and also in her own ability to identify patient problems and give effective nursing care.

Such then are the benefits which accrue to individual nurses caring for groups of patients. In what way is the nursing process of advantage to the ward sister or nurse in change of a ward? The identification of patient problems and their requirements for nursing care provides the ward sister with some indication of the work load generated by each patient. In addition the ward sister is also able to identify the levels of skill and knowledge required by nurses to undertake the nursing care required by patients. With this information the ward sister is better placed to delegate patient care according to work load and levels of skill necessary. Used in this way the nursing process becomes a tool for ward management as well as a tool for the management of individual patient care.

We are aware that the use of the nursing care plan is a means of communication. Such written communication of nursing care required by patients has the potential of easing the burden of ward sisters of the constant interruptions to which they are so often subjected. In addition, the freedom from constant interruption permits the ward sister time to supervise and teach nurse learners as they plan and implement nursing care. This potential for increased contact time between nurse learners and ward sister enables the latter to assess more readily the nurse learners' learning needs and progress during their experience on the ward.

The actual process of identifying patient problems and planning care provides an ideal opportunity for teaching. The use of the nursing care plan and the nursing care planning conference has previously been discussed in this respect. It is one more example of the way in which the nursing process can be used to advantage.

However, in addition to providing the ward sisters with an opportunity to evaluate nurse learners' progress, they are also able to evaluate patient progress in relation to the care which has been given. Yet another type of evaluation is possible: with the information available from the nursing care plans and patient progress notes, the ward sisters may evaluate the effectiveness of their organisation of resources.

Did the ward sister correctly match the needs of patients for care with the levels of skill of the nurses? Is there any particular item of equipment frequently used that might be requested for the ward? Does reviewing patients' nursing care plans demonstrate any particular pattern of work load? If so, might this be considered when planning the nurses' duty rota?

While the latter discussion has focussed on advantages for the nursing staff, it will be evident that these advantages are also indirectly beneficial to the patient.

References and Suggested Further Readings

Bergman, R. (1974) Typology for teamwork – Way of determining who should be on a specific nursing or health care team in varying situations. *Am. J. of Nursing*, Vol. 74, No. 9 (September 1974), pp. 1618–20.

Duberley, J. (1977) Talking Point: How will the change strike you and me. *Nursing Times*, Vol. 73, No. 45 (10 November 1977), pp. 1736–39.

Kron, T. (1976) *The Management of Patient Care*. Philadelphia: W. B. Saunders Co.

Lewis, L. C. (1970) *Planning Patient Care*. Dubuque, Iowa: W. C. Brown Co.

Marks-Maran, D. (1978) Patient allocation v. task allocation in relation to the nursing process. *Nursing Times*, Vol. 74 (9 March 1978), pp. 413–16.

Marriner, A. (1975) *The Nursing Process*. In A scientific approach to nursing care. St. Louis: C. V. Mosby.

Mayers, M. (1978) *A Systematic Approach to the Nursing Care Plan*, 2nd ed. New York: Appleton-Century-Crofts Ltd.

Norton, D. (1970) *By Accident or Design?* Edinburgh: Churchill-Livingstone.

Pembrey, S. (1975) From work routines to patient assignment. An experiment in ward organisation. (A change from task to patient assignment). *Nursing Times*, Vol. 71, No. 45 (6 November 1975), pp. 1768–72.

Sharp, B. H. & E. Cross (1971) Rounds and rounds. (Nursing team rounds for patient care planning). *Nursing Outlook*, Vol. 9, No. 6 (June 1971). pp. 419–20.

Tatton Brown, W. (1978) Owed to the Nightingale. An assessment of ward design. *Nursing Times*, Vol. 74, No. 31 (3 August 1978), pp. 1273–78.

—— (1978) Owed to the Nightingale – 2: Ward evaluation. A review of three types of ward at St. Thomas'. *Ibid.*, pp. 1279–84.

Varga (1973) Symposium on the management and supervision of patient care. *Nursing Clinics of North America*. Vol. 8, No. 2 (June 1973), pp. 203–373.

—— (1974) The nurse-doctor relationship. *Nursing Times*, Vol. 70 (10 January 1974), pp. 44–48.

5. Evaluating Nursing Care

Evaluation, as part of the nursing process, has been a much neglected area of study and has not been well documented; hence nurses have been deprived of the opportuntiy of becoming familiar with the concept and as a result often think of it as difficult. Our aim is to present the principles of evaluation of nursing care as simply and as logically as possible in an attempt to encourage nurses to become more objective and creative in their care-giving role. Examples are given for a clearer understanding of the evaluative component of the nursing process.

Assessment, planning and action without evaluation cannot provide us with the information we need to improve practice and hence the quality of patient care.

What is Evaluation?

Broadly speaking, evaluation is concerned with measuring the effectiveness of nursing care; this incorporates the concept of change. Nurses are constantly involved in assessing changes in a patient's condition. Discussed in terms of measurement of change, evaluation can seem difficult, however we are already involved in this process and need only to become more aware of it. There are very few established devices for measuring changes in a patient's condition in nursing, but there is one instrument that every nurse is familiar with and that is the clinical thermometer. We constantly use the clinical thermometer to evaluate the nursing care which we give to patients who have either a high or low body temperature. A simple example illustrating how we are already involved with evaluation would be:

A twenty-three-year-old woman has a temperature of 39.5°C at 10 A.M. The nursing action instituted as a result of the raised body temperature is to take the blankets off the bed and to place a cold air fan at the bedside. It is expected that by 11 A.M. the patient's temperature should have fallen to 39°C. The means of measuring whether the nursing care has been effective is to retake the patient's temperature.

If we have asked ourselves the question:

How do I know that the nursing care I give is assisting the patient in his recovery?

we have already begun to think about change, measurement, effectiveness and evaluation. Thinking about the appropriateness and the effectiveness of nursing care is a good starting point from which to look at evaluation in greater depth.

Assessment and Evaluation

Evaluation bears some relationship to assessment; both involve the collection of information. The data collected during the assessment stage of the nursing process are of a more general nature than the information collected during the evaluation stage and are used as a data base from which patient problems can be identified. The data collected for evaluation purposes are specific to the criteria inherent in each patient goal. Assessment and evaluation are ongoing processes and can occur wherever and whenever a nurse is in contact with a patient. Although assessment is the first stage in the nursing process and evaluation the last they can occur almost simultaneously. Examples of this are given later.

The nurse uses the same skills to collect the data for assessment and evaluation. These skills are

1. observation	4. cueing
2. interviewing	5. inference
3. record-searching	6. interpretation
	7. consultation

Although the skills used by the nurse are the same in assessment and evaluation there is one fundamental difference between these two stages. Evaluation can be carried out only after the patient goals have been set and some nursing action has been undertaken to achieve the goal. The assessment provides the information necessary to identify patient problems and these problems should be validated wherever possible. Evaluation relates to the effectiveness of the nursing care given to alleviate the actual or potential patient problem. In short, evaluation is only possible after the patient goal has been made explicit and can only take place after we have provided care.

Statement of Patient Goals

Statement A. The patient will drink more fluid.

In statement *A* the patient goal appears clear at first glance. However, we have to ask ourselves what we understand by the word *more*. More than what amount and over what period of time should we evaluate the care. We have to decide how much more we wish the patient to drink and for how long. Statement *A* is not a well-formulated statement of a patient goal because each nurse can interpret it in a different way.

Statement B. The patient will drink 3,000 ml of fluid in twenty-four hours.

Statement *B* is a better formulated statement of a goal. We are left in no doubt; the patient's fluid intake should be 3,000 ml in twenty-four hours. If we look more closely at this statement it can be seen to be ambiguous; 3,000 ml is the amount of fluid that the patient is required to drink in a twenty-four-hour period. However, it is doubtful if the patient will actually receive the amount, because no mention has been made of the amount of fluid the patient is to drink each hour and no allowance has been made for the time that the patient is asleep.

Statement C. The patient will drink 200 ml of fluid each hour between 7 A.M. and 10 P.M. (totalling 3,000 ml in twenty-four hours).

Statement *C* is clearly written, it is unambiguous and an allowance has been made for the time the patient is usually asleep. The patient is to drink 200 ml of fluid each hour between 7 A.M. and 10 P.M. The goal is flexible in that the total amount for the day is stated as 3,000 ml, so if the patient wakes later and goes to sleep later an adjustment can be made accordingly. It is anticipated that if a nurse followed the instructions inherent in this goal the patient would receive 3,000 ml of fluid in twenty-four hours. To carry out the evaluation it would be necessary to measure the fluid drunk each hour by the patient and to record it accurately on a fluid balance chart.

The Five Stages in Evaluation

There are five stages in the evaluation process; they are

1. The selection of observable criteria related to the desired patient goal
2. The collection of relevant information
3. A comparison of the information collected with the selected criteria
4. A judgement about the patient's response reflected by the comparison; this involves the concept of change
5. Feedback and modification of the Nursing Care Plan.

Selection of Observable Criteria Related to the Desired Patient Goal

The statements of desired patient goals are set in relation to the actual and potential problems identified and validated during the assessment stage of the nursing process. (It may be helpful here to reread the chapter on Assessment.)

Validation of patient problems and evaluation

Validation in the context of the nursing process requires us to confirm that the problems identified during the assessment phase are recognised as problems by the patient. The ratification of the problems' existence to the patient is important but not absolutely essential. Validation is useful because if patients recognise the problem they can be involved more readily in the nursing care plan. This then makes care planning a joint exercise between the nurse and the patient.

It is not possible to validate the existence of all problems with the patient, although every attempt should be made to do so. In some situations the patient will lack the professional knowledge necessary to recognise a problem. This is sometimes more apparent when dealing with potential problems. An elderly person may have no knowledge of hypothermia and fail to recognise it as a potential problem. Problems of slow onset are also difficult to validate with patients. A hearing loss of gradual onset may be confirmed by audiometric tests but be denied by the patient as a problem.

Validation is largely concerned with confirming that the patient is aware of the problem's existence. If the patient is unaware of the problem it may be necessary to set additional goals (examples are given). Evaluation, on the other hand, is concerned with measuring the effectiveness of nursing care and unlike validation it can only be carried out after nursing action has been undertaken. Validation of a patient's problem enters into evaluation in two ways:

1. It affects the nurse's choice in determining criteria inherent in the patient goal statements.

2. If the evaluation of nursing care is to be subjective the nurse may confirm with the patient that a change has taken place.

We are already aware that actual patient problems are sometimes more easily validated than potential problems. A patient with an existing pressure sore will usually acknowledge the sore as a problem which requires nursing action and will tolerate the nursing care involved, such as two hourly turning throughout the night in order to facilitate healing. However, a patient who is at risk from developing pressure sores according to the Norton Pressure Sore Risk Assessment Scale (see Table 1) may not accept this as a potential problem requiring preventive nursing action. As a result he may complain bitterly about his two hourly turns, especially during the night.

Table 1.–**Pressure Sore Risk Assessment**

A		B		C		D		E	
Physical condition		*Mental condition*		*Activity*		*Mobility*		*Incontinent*	
Good	4	Alert	4	Ambulant	4	Full	4	Not	4
Fair	3	Apathetic	3	Walk/help	3	Slightly limited	3	Occasionally	3
Poor	2	Confused	2	Chairbound	2	Very limited	2	Usually/urine	2
Very bad	1	Stuporous	1	Bedfast	1	Immobile	1	Doubly	1

Key: Total score of 14 or below = 'at risk' (pressure sore risk assessment form. (Norton, et al. (1962) *Report: An Investigation of Geriatric Nursing Problems in Hospital*. Edinburgh: Churchill-Livingstone

In the case of the patient who has the potential problem of likelihood of developing pressure sores we may set additional goals. An example of additional goals for a patient at risk would be:

A. 11/6/79   The patient will say that he understands why he is turned two hourly throughout the night by 10 P.M. on the 12/6/79.

B. 12/6/79   The patient will tolerate being turned during the night and will indicate this by no longer shouting by 10 P.M. 13/6/79.

Examples *A* and *B* would be goal statements appropriate for a patient who was capable of speaking; whereas example *B* statement could be used for a patient who was not capable of speaking as in the case of a person who had suffered a cerebral vascular accident which had affected the speech centre.

Formulation of patient goals

Patient goals *must* be clearly stated and should incorporate a time element. If a patient is on a reducing diet it is not enough to say: The patient will lose weight. A realistic target weight should be set wherever possible. For example,

21/6/79   10 A.M.   The patient will lose 1 kg in body weight by 10 A.M. 28/6/79

In some situations it is not possible to formulate a well-defined goal statement and here a broad goal statement has to take its place. The patient with a pressure sore is a good example. It is possible to measure the patient's pressure sore and to describe the appearance of the tissue and this could be stated as:

A patient is admitted to hospital with a sacral pressure sore. The sore measures 2 cm in width, 3 cm in length and 0.5 cm in depth at its deepest point. The tissue appears inflamed and there is pus in the sore.

The pressure sore is measured with a ruler and a probe is used to measure the depth of the sore at its deepest point. The tissue is described as it appears to the nurse, and the presence of infection can be confirmed by taking a swab for bacteriological culture. The statement of the patient goal cannot be specific enough to indicate the size of reduction expected in the pressure sore, because the nursing profession, as yet, does not have the knowledge to predict the size of pressure sore reduction in relation to treatment over time. However, it is hoped that if nurses record the actual size of the sore at each evaluation, information will eventually be available to allow us to be more specific in setting patient goals. Despite the fact that we cannot predict the size of the reduction in the pressure sore there are two broad goals. An example of a statement of patient goals is:

A. The pressure sore should show a continuing reduction in size until completely healed.
B. The tissue should show signs of reduction in the amount of infection.

The way the nurse will know if the infection is less is by the amount of visible pus and inflamed tissue. This can be confirmed by taking a swab for culture. Examples *A* and *B* are, however, in their present form meaningless because the element of time has not been included. Clearly it is more desirable for the patient goal to be achieved in a week rather than a month or a year. The goal statements do not give a firm evaluation date and are therefore open-ended. It would have been better if the goals read:

A. 19/6/79   10 A.M. The pressure sore should show a reduction in size by 10 A.M. 26/6/79.
B. 19/6/79   10 A.M. The tissue should show signs of a reduction in the amount of infection by 10 A.M. 26/6/79.

In the second example of the goal statements there is the date the statement was made and the date the evaluation is to be carried out. If the desired goal is not achieved in seven days we may continue the treatment and set another evaluation date, we may decide to change the treatment and set another evaluation date, or alternatively we may modify the patient goal and set another evaluation date. By placing a time limit on evaluation it enables us to examine the care we give in relation to the patient's progress, and provides an opportunity to change the care plan. If no time limit is imposed information relating to the patient goal may not be recorded and the nursing profession may not acquire the information it needs to predict the outcome of nursing care.

Because formal evaluative dates have been advocated this is not intended to deter us from evaluating the progress of the patient away or towards his goal more frequently. The evaluation date merely formalises the process and acts as a reminder to those who may not be in the habit of evaluating the care they give, or recording the evaluation to do so. Similarly if a patient's condition suddenly changes it may be necessary to alter the evaluation criteria and dates. The selection of observable criteria is crucial to the evaluation process. In the examples given weight was an observable criterion measurable in kilograms or pounds and ounces on scales. The reduction in size of a pressure sore is measurable by using a ruler and can be measured in millimetres and the reduction of infection can be estimated visually by the reduction of inflamed tissue and the amount of pus present. This may be confirmed by bacteriological investigations. The amount of fluid consumed by a patient can be measured in millilitres.

The Collection of Relevant Information
During the assessment phase of the nursing process, information is systematically collected in a variety of areas, that is, physical, social, psychological and spiritual. In evaluating nursing care it is only necessary to collect information related to the statement of the desired patient goal. The examples given so far in this chapter have been easy to understand because the way the change in the patient condition was to be measured has been concrete. There has been an instrument available which has made the comparison objective. However, not all patient goals are measurable in terms of quantifiable amounts such as size, weight or degrees. Many changes in patients are much more elusive and involve the observation and interpretation of behavioural cues. The subtle differences in behaviour may be illustrated by thinking in general terms of a patient who has undergone surgery which has resulted in the formation of a stoma. After the immediate postoperative period the broad aim of nursing care is usually to help the patient adjust psychologically to living with a stoma and to help the patient to manage the practical care of the stoma. The way we teach the patient to cope with the practical management of the stoma varies according to the patient's physical and psychological capabilities.

The goal statements for different patients should indicate the various ways in which the same goal is to be reached. One of the important goal statements relating to a patient who has undergone surgery resulting in a stoma may be:

20/6/79   The patient will be able to change his or her own stoma bag whenever necessary before discharge from hospital.

This is a broad goal statement. It is often necessary to break a goal down into a series of stages, or subgoals, in order to identify criteria or specific behavioural cues which may be interpreted as movement away from or towards the desired goal. There are many ways in which patients can react to major surgery involving mutilation of a part of the body and a number of factors which could be said to influence their reaction. Age, sex, marital status, intelligence level, prognosis and past experience of hospital or illness all exert influence on the way in which a patient reacts after surgery. One would expect a single girl, aged 25 years, engaged to be married, who enjoys sport and works as a sales assistant to experience different problems in coming to terms with a stoma than an independent elderly widower with rheumatoid arthritis of the hands. These two examples are taken further to illustrate the problems experienced by each patient which lead to the setting of different patient goals.

A. Five days after the operation Jane, a 25-year-old patient, is very withdrawn and refuses to talk to the nurses. She closes her eyes whenever her dressing is changed and cries frequently.

In this case it is necessary to break the ultimate goal of the patient caring for her own stoma down into a series of intermediate goals, or subgoals, in an attempt to identify the behaviour we should expect which will demonstrate whether the patient is moving away from or towards the ultimate goal.

Example of Intermediate Goals, or Subgoals
1/7/78   A.M. The patient will talk to the nurse.
2/7/78   A.M. The patient will talk about herself to the nurse.
2/7/78   P.M. The patient will talk about her hospitalization to the nurse.
3/7/78   A.M. The patient will talk about her operation to the nurse.
3/7/78   P.M. The patient will engage in conversation and keep her eyes open while her dressing is changed.
4/7/78   A.M. The patient will allow the nurse to talk to her about the way the stoma functions.

4/7/78 P.M. The patient will look at and hold a clean stoma bag.

5/7/78 A.M. The patient will look at her stoma while the bag is changed.

5/7/78 P.M. The patient will assist the nurse in changing the stoma bag.

6/7/78 A.M. The patient will assist the nurse in changing the stoma bag.

6/7/78 P.M. The patient will allow the nurse to assist her in changing the bag.

7/7/78 A.M. The patient will change the bag herself under the supervision of the nurse.

7/7/78 P.M. The patient will change the bag herself under the supervision of the nurse.

8/7/78 A.M. The patient will change the bag herself with no supervision.

The preceding goal statements convey to us the behaviour we are to look for and the information to be collected about the patient. In the example, both verbal and non-verbal behaviour are observed and are equally important in evaluating how far the patient has moved both physically and psychologically towards the ultimate goal of caring for her own stoma. Not many nurses have the time to write down all the intermediary goals and this is not essential. Much of the information that nurses collect in connection with intermediary goals is often reported in a formal ward report session or is handed on at the change of shift.

The goals have been written here to emphasise that the nurse is not just waiting for the patient to be able to change her own stoma bag but plans the nursing care to encourage the patient to move towards the goal as soon as possible. It is important that goal and intermediary goal statements whenever possible are observable; the ultimate goal in this case is observable. The patient can be seen to change her own stoma bag. There are other behaviours as indicated in the subgoal statements that we will interpret as the patient moves towards the desired goal. If the patient does not move quickly enough towards the goal we may change our intervention. Subgoal statements are important but should perhaps be regarded as part of the mental process which we undergo to identify which cues to look for to determine how far the patient has moved towards the ultimate goal, in this case changing a stoma bag. It is important to state the patient goal clearly, and if possible to indicate the criteria we are to use to evaluate the care we give.

> *B.* Mr Jones is an independent elderly widower with rheumatoid arthritis of the hands and on the tenth postoperative day he is concerned about how he is going to manage his colostomy at home.

The major problem for Mr Jones is that owing to his arthritis he does not have the manual dexterity needed to manage his colostomy. Psychologically he appears to have adjusted to the stoma but he is physically incapable of managing his own colostomy. The care Mr Jones receives from the nurse and the problems he experiences in relation to his stoma are very different from those of Jane. The intermediate goal or subgoal statements for Mr Jones might read:

> 27/7/78   A.M. The patient will try to use another brand of colostomy bag.
> 27/7/78   P.M. The patient will talk to the nurse when she changes the bag of his worries in relation to discharge.
> 28/7/78   A.M. The patient will talk about the district nurse coming to visit him daily when he goes home.
> 28/7/78   P.M. The patient will indicate his acceptance of the district nurse visiting him at home and expresses a desire to go home.
> 29/7/78   A.M. The patient will express a desire to meet the district nurse prior to discharge from hospital.

The major problem for Mr Jones has been to give up some of his independence and allow himself to become dependent on the nurse to change his colostomy bag. The care Jane and Mr Jones needed was different although their condition was similar in that they were both patients who had surgery for the formation of a stoma. The broad goal for each patient was the same; however, the evaluation criteria were different as indicated in the subgoal statements. The evaluation criteria were patient specific and not condition specific. Jane achieved her ultimate goal, Mr Jones did not, prior to discharge from hospital.

A Comparison of the Information collected with the Selected Criteria

After the patient goal has been stated the evaluation criteria are selected. The information to be collected in the evaluation process is guided by the selected criteria; subjective data and objective data are reflected in the criteria. We collect the information using our full range of skills. Information related to the nurse by the patient is referred to as subjective data. For example,

The patient said that he slept well last night.

Information obtained by observing the patient's behaviour is referred to as objective data. Then,

The nurse observed the patient six times during the night, his breathing was deep and regular, he was lying on his side, his eyes were closed and he did not respond to his name.

The nurse infers from the cues, regular deep breathing, closed eyes, and not responding to his name on six occasions that the patient slept well during the night. This is objective data.

Evaluation is dependent upon the comparison of information collected before nursing action has been taken with information collected after nursing action has been taken. It is this comparison which makes evaluation different, otherwise it could be referred to as reassessment. We are already aware that the skills used in evaluation to collect data are the same as those used in assessment; however the data collected in the evaluation are determined by the selected criteria and are not of a general nature, as in the assessment phase.

The information collected at the initial assessment of the patient provides the base-line data for comparison. In this respect assessment and evaluation are ongoing, assessment becomes evaluation when the element of comparison is introduced. Let us look at another example, as it is important to have a clear understanding of the concept of evaluation in relation to assessment.

A pressure sore size 2 cm long, 1 cm wide and 0.5 cm deep is identified during the assessment process.

The goal is set as a continuous reduction in size of the pressure sore.

The evaluation date is set at weekly intervals until the sore is completely healed.

The selected criterion is size and is measurable using a ruler and probe.

At the assessment we measured the pressure sore using a ruler and a probe and found its dimensions to be 2 cm × 1 cm × 0.5 cm. At the evaluation a week later we did the same and found its size to be 2 cm × 1 cm × 0.5 cm. We compared the second measurement with the measurement taken at the assessment and found that there had been no change in the size of the pressure sore. The actions we carried out on both occasions were identical, the difference was that in the evaluation we compared the second measurement to the measurement identified in the assessment. If the measurement had been smaller or larger on the evaluation date this would have told us that there had been a favourable or unfavourable change.

The measurements, in this example, at the first evaluation date were identical indicating no change; at subsequent evaluations the measurements may be different. Evaluation is ongoing, in that, each time a patient problem is evaluated the result is recorded so it is not always necessary, for example, to compare the pressure sore size with the size of the sore at the assessment. The assessment always provides the base line, but it is often easier to compare the size with the preceding evaluation measurement. This means that the nurse has some understanding of the meaning of the change. Here the pressure sore was the same size 2 cm × 1 cm × 0.5 cm at the first evaluation as it was at the assessment. If it had increased in size to 2.5 cm long by 1.5 cm wide and 0.5 cm depth it would be most important to compare the second evaluation to the first because once a change has occurred it outdates the initial information.

Not all evaluation takes place over a long time period. Evaluation can take place almost immediately.

A nurse goes to a patient to take his temperature. She puts the thermometer in his mouth and leaves it for three minutes when she takes it out. It reads, 38°C. This could be equated with assessment; the nurse assesses that the patient's temperature is 38°C. She then compares the patient's temperature of 38°C to the expected normal for an oral body temperature which is 37°C and concludes that the patient has a temperature 1°C above the expected normal. This is evaluation which has involved comparison and has taken place within the span of half a minute.

Very few nurses have really thought that when they take a patient's temperature they are making an evaluation but that is what we are doing. We are comparing the patient's temperature to the expected normal and act upon the information and may change the nursing action accordingly.

After the nursing action has been carried out another comparison can be made. In the case of a patient with a raised body temperature a fan or tepid sponging may be the action of choice. After half an hour the nurse may retake the patient's temperature and make two comparisons: the first, with the most recent reading on the TPR chart and, the second, with the normal body temperature. Most temperature charts allow visual comparison and there is a continuous line drawn at the expected normal body temperature.

The evaluation of a patient's temperature involved explicit measurement and is referred to as objective data. We know that subjective data are also important. An example showing where subjective data are used in evaluation would be:

A nurse observes that a patient looks uncomfortable.

This is objective data. The nurse will then pick up cues such as that the patient's posture looks abnormal, the neck is extended and not supported. She infers from this that the patient is uncomfortable. She validates this by asking the patient if he is comfortable. If the patient says he is not comfortable this then validates the problem. The nurse intervenes by rearranging the pillows and evaluates her own performance by asking the patient if he is comfortable. *This* is subjective data but is a reliable way of evaluating. In this instance it was the patient who made the comparison, he compared the way he felt before the pillows were moved to the way he felt afterwards.

The nurse could do her own evaluation by comparing the patient's posture before and after the pillows were moved. This would be objective data. Such episodes happen many times a day on any hospital ward and the assessment and evaluation together take as little as thirty seconds. The nurse would not be expected to record this type of information and indeed would not have time to do so, but she would be expected to record any abnormal or unexpected information. If a patient looked uncomfortable in bed and was found on closer examination to have a weakness on one side of his body which was not there previously the nurse would be expected to record this.

The patient is important in evaluating nursing action and should always be consulted. If it is not possible to collect objective data it is nearly always possible to collect subjective data which if used for comparative purposes can be quite informative and should not be underestimated. If objective data can be collected alongside subjective data this strengthens the evaluation but the absence of objective data should not be used as an excuse for not evaluating nursing care.

Judgement and Decision-making

After we have collected the relevant information and compared it with the selected evaluative criteria to determine if there has been a change in the patient's condition a decision has to be made.

The primary concern of evaluation is to find out if the nursing care given has been effective in achieving the patient goal and alleviating the patient problem, or in preventing a potential problem from developing. There are three possible outcomes in evaluation:

1. The stated patient goal has been achieved by or on the evaluation date.

2. The stated patient goal has not been achieved by or on the evaluation date.

3. The stated patient goal has been partially achieved by or on the evaluation date.

Unfortunately inherent in the evaluation process is the possibility of three types of error.

1. If a patient achieves his goal we have to ask ourselves if we set the goal too low and we must use our professional judgement to decide at what level to set the goal.

2. Alternatively if the patient does not achieve his goal we must ask ourselves if we set the goal too high.

3. If the patient only partially achieves his goal by the evaluation date we must judge if the evaluation date and the goal were appropriate to the patient.

Decision-making is a complex process and necessitates a choice from many alternatives. Nurses should be able to judge which alternative to choose. We may do this by identifying a list of choices from the most desirable through to the least desirable. There are several constraints which influence the choice of alternatives before a decision is made:

1. the number of choices we can think of depends on our knowledge and previous experience
2. the number of nurses or others involved in the care of the patient
3. the amount of time available
4. the resources of the hospital/ward

Before a choice is made the nurse should compare all the alternatives with each other in order to select the best one. She should consider the consequences of each alternative for every action, for there is usually more than one outcome. The nurse should decide the probability or likelihood of a goal being achieved. The area of probability cannot yet be well defined because in nursing we do not yet have the knowledge to predict accurately likely outcomes following certain nursing actions. We can only hope to accumulate this knowledge by evaluating patient care.

If at the evaluation it is found that the patient has not moved either away or towards the goal we have to make a decision. We have a choice of four alternatives:

1. change the goal, keep treatment the same
2. change the treatment, keep the goal the same
3. change the goal and treatment
4. change the evaluation date and keep treatment and goal the same

How do we decide what to do? At present the only answer is to claim that the nurse uses her professional judgement in order to make her decision. However, professional judgement is based on knowledge and so the nurse uses her knowledge of nursing and the sciences which underlie it together with her past experience to help her decide which alternative to choose. The judgement she makes will vary among patients, because patients vary among themselves.

Evaluation can only be useful if the findings are acted upon. The quality of patient care can be improved by nurses appraising the care they give and altering it accordingly. At the present time we do not have the information available to predict the outcome of nursing care for every patient but it is hoped that if we evaluate the care we give and change our: goal statement; nursing actions; or evaluation criteria/date, then we will as a profession accumulate sufficient data to predict with moderate accuracy the likelihood of each patient response in relation to the nursing action performed for a stated patient problem.

Feedback and Modification of the Care Plan

The nursing care plan is discussed in detail in chapter 3. It is enough to say here that the nurse should change the care plan in accordance with her decision based on the comparison of data before and after nursing action, which indicates how far the patient has moved towards his goal. Even if no changes are made in the treatment or goal, the date the evaluation was carried out and the result should be recorded.

We are aware that certain information need not be recorded on the care plan. The example given was the adjustment of a patient's pillows involving evaluation of the patient's comfort. There is no explicit rule regarding information which should be and should not be recorded on the care plan and rules are often determined by hospital or ward policy. The term *care plan* is used but this also refers to the plans of care written in the nursing Kardex or in other record books. As a basic rule to follow, a problem should only be recorded if it is intended to take action on it. Similarly after evaluation, if a problem is resolved, an alteration should be made on the plan, also any changes in the desired goal or evaluation date should be recorded.

Updating of care plans can usually be done once a day, though it may be necessary in acute areas such as intensive care units to update the plan more frequently. Any changes to care plans should be brought to the attention of nurses at the change of shift report. Approved abbreviations may be used. However, it is not advisable for nurses to use their own abbreviations since confusion may result if abbreviations are misinterpreted. Evaluation of nursing care provides the necessary feedback to update the care plan and the impetus to change nursing action.

Evaluation is often neglected because we sometimes feel that it takes too long and we would rather concentrate on giving patient care than on evaluating the effects of the care we have given. However, it is worth remembering that if we wish to improve the quality of nursing care generally then we need to evaluate the care we give to individual patients.

The Nursing Process and Formal Auditing of Patient Records

The nursing process is a problem-solving approach to patient care and involves the systematic recording of a patient's progress to enable evaluation in terms of patient-goal attainment to take place. The accurate recording of a patient's progress also enables the process of patient care to be examined or audited.

The audit takes place retrospectively after the patient has been discharged from hospital. Auditing after discharge is thought to give an over-all view of the total nursing care which a patient received during his stay in hospital as reflected in the patient records. The patient's records include charts, the nursing Kardex and care plan. There are, however, inherent difficulties in using records for evaluation purposes, the most obvious being that the quality of record keeping may be evaluated instead of the care the patient received.

The Evaluative Aspect of Auditing

Evaluation implies comparison. In auditing the base line for comparison is provided by a set of predetermined standards agreed upon by the organisation, hospital or community division carrying out the audit. Essentially nursing audit is a tool of management. It is the divisional nursing officer or senior manager who has the ultimate responsibility for the over-all quality of nursing care in a hospital. It is therefore a management decision to implement the use of audit. Before this decision is taken the full cooperation of the nursing staff is needed, because if the patients' records are to be evaluated to see if the care they received met the predetermined standards then the records must contain relevant information. Systematic recording as in the problem oriented approach to record keeping is a prerequisite to the introduction of nursing audit.

Auditing appears to identify the weak links in the nursing process and can generate interesting topics for continuing nurse education. As anything other than a management tool the nursing audit has shortcomings. The audit is carried out after the patient has been discharged from hospital so there is no reasonable way in which care can be improved for an individual patient. Auditing is thought to improve record keeping because we become more discriminating in our recording since we know it may be evaluated.

In contrast to the audit, individual patient-goal-attainment evaluation can be carried out by every nurse and there is an opportunity to modify and improve upon the care given to any patient. Evaluation as part of the nursing process referred to here as goal-attainment evaluation is the province of the clinical nurse and can be acted upon by her.

Informal Auditing of Patient Records

The word *audit*, according to The Concise Oxford Dictionary, means to 'examine officially'. The official examination of patient's nursing records has been referred to as formal auditing and this is usually considered to be a management function. The ward sister or staff nurse may wish to examine past nursing records in a less formal way and this approach has been referred to as informal auditing.

Probably the most common reason for a ward sister or staff nurse wishing to examine retrospectively patients' nursing records would be either for research purposes or to verify a hunch or intuition. For example,

A ward sister may think that patients who receive extra fluids rather than a specific mouth-care procedure are less likely to develop mouth ulcers. If the nursing records have been kept in a systematic way, they will reflect the stages of the nursing process. It should therefore be possible, firstly, to identify the patients who received either extra fluids or a specific mouth-care procedure for a similar problem, and, secondly, it should be possible to isolate those patients who developed mouth ulcers. This information would allow the ward sister to verify or refute her hunch.

At the present time in nursing we know very little about factors which can be used to predict patient outcomes in relation to specific problems and nursing actions. By looking back over patients' records after they have been discharged from hospital it may be possible to identify factors related to variables, such as age, sex, marital status and ethnic group, which might help nurses in predicting the probability of certain patient outcomes occurring in relation to specified problems and actions.

Informal auditing does not involve a comparison against predetermined standards; however, it still has implications for nursing practice at ward level and potential implications for the professional development of nursing.

The Nursing Care Plan: An Instrument of Evaluation

The nursing care plan can be used by us to evaluate our own performance in terms of whether the patient achieved his stated goal. Self-evaluation although difficult is advocated as a means of improving standards of nursing care. To participate in self-evaluation we would need to be very determined and conscientious, since it is difficult if we find that the care we give is not being effective to acknowledge the fact and do something positive about it and it is rather more easy to abandon evaluation altogether.

The nursing care plan incorporating a column for documentation of rationale for nursing action can be used by nurse tutors to evaluate a learner's progress. The learner would be required to assess a patient, identify his problem and to plan his subsequent care, documenting the reasons why she planned the specific care. This is referred to as 'the rationale for nursing action'. The tutor over time would expect to see an extension of the learner's knowledge reflected in the problem identified, care planned and rationale.

The nursing care plan reflecting a problem-solving approach to nursing care can be used by learners to evaluate each other's progress. This is referred to as 'peer evaluation'. Learners would be required to present a case study of a patient whom they had nursed. The case study would be expected to include a summary of the patient's problems, the care plan and rationale for action and patient outcome in terms of goal attainment. The learner group would then discuss the care given in relation to the rationale and outcome and put forward alternative approaches and rationale. It is hoped that this would highlight the strengths and weaknesses of the presented plan.

Evaluation of Nursing Care: An Experiment

Evaluative experiments in nursing are now becoming more acceptable. It is useful for nurses to come to terms with the principles of evaluation and to use them as a means of developing effective and efficient care.

Most nurses at one time or another have had thoughts about nursing care X being more effective than care Y in a given situation. Their ideas or suspicions are rarely followed through, but should be if nursing practice is to improve. Many nurses have thought of one nursing procedure as more effective than another in certain situations, for example, in preventing or treating pressure sores or providing mouth care.

> A nurse may have an intuition that treatment X is more effective than treatment Y for preventing pressure sores on the heels of elderly patients. This intuition raises a question:
> Does treatment X work better than treatment Y in preventing pressure sores on the heels?

The nurse can find out the answer to the question by conducting a clinical experiment.

A clinical experiment

The experiment is to find out if treatment X is more effective than treatment Y in preventing pressure sores on the heels of elderly patients.

Treatment X is using sheepskin bootees when the patient is in bed and treatment Y is massaging the heels twice a day. The nurse had a feeling that treatment X worked better than treatment Y. She thought that more patients had pressure sores on their heels after receiving treatment Y. However a nurse cannot change the treatment on the ward on the basis of a hunch. It is necessary to obtain proof, to demonstrate which treatment is more effective. A hypothetical experiment using the example already given is:

> It was agreed among the ward staff to allow the experiment to continue for three months. It was decided that which ever treatment was more effective in preventing pressure sores on the heels would be the treatment of choice on the ward after the experiment. Each new admission to the ward was included in

the experiment, if they were at risk from developing pressure sores according to the Norton Pressure Sore Assessment Scale. Each patient was given both treatment X and treatment Y. This could be done because the interest was in the prevention of pressure sores on the heels and all the patients in the study had two heels. The right heel was used for treatment X and the foot was marked with a cross on the sole to remind the nurses. The left heel was used for treatment Y. The patients received the experimental treatment to both heels until they were discharged or transferred from the ward or were no longer at risk from developing pressure sores. The condition of each patient's heels was recorded daily by the nurse caring for the patient and at the end of three months the number of pressure sores which developed on the heels was recorded and a comparison was made between the right heel, treatment X, and the left heel, treatment Y.

The experiment seems quite straightforward. However, there will always be some problems in conducting an experiment. In this one the major problem would be gaining the support of all the nursing staff so that they would carry out the treatment according to the rules of the experiment.

There are a number of everyday nursing procedures which would lend themselves nicely to comparative experimentation. Mouth care or oral hygiene is a much debated topic. Are extra fluids more effective at keeping a patient's mouth clean and moist than specific oral hygiene routines?

Many clinical experiments are the result of hunches which nurses have and which generate questions to be answered. Here a simple experiment has been shown which is probably within the capabilities of every nurse. We hope that thinking of evaluation in these terms will inspire us to search for answers to questions which are currently in our mind regarding the effectiveness of certain types of nursing care. Evaluation of patient care in terms of goal attainment or experimentation with different types of nursing care in relation to specific goals as in the X–Y example are ways of finding out more about nursing and improving the care given to patients. There are many problems which need to be solved in nursing and it is hoped that evaluation *will* inspire nurses to seek the answers to some of the many questions which remain unanswered.

References and Suggested Further Readings

Chrisp, M. (1977) New treatment for pressure sores. *Nursing Times*, Vol.73, No. 31 (4 August 1977), pp. 1202–5.

Howarth, H. (1977) Mouth care procedures for the very ill. *Nursing Times*, Vol. 73, No. 10 (10 March 1977), pp. 354–5.

Norton, D. et al. (1975) *An Investigation of Geriatric Nursing Problems in Hospital.* Reprint. Edinburgh: Churchill-Livingstone.

Rhodes, B. et al. (1979) The treatment of pressure sores in geriatric patients: A trial of Sterculia powder. *Nursing Times*, Vol. 75, No. 9 (1 March 1979), pp. 365–8.

6. Community Care

So far we have discussed the nursing process in general terms, and have looked at its use in a variety of hospital settings. Our purpose in this has been twofold. We have been trying to demonstrate that the basic assumptions of the nursing process are always the same: to use the process is simply a way of being logical and beginning at the beginning by assessing a particular patient's needs as a basis for planning and giving his care and finishing by asking whether our assessment and plans were successful as judged by results. It should also be obvious that this end was not really an end at all, but a starting point for either reassessing and replanning that particular patient's care, or as a basis for improving the care of future patients. On the other hand, all these immutable parts of the process are affected by our fundamental appreciation of what we think nursing is – whether we think it is a paramedical occupation concerned mainly with carrying out doctors' orders or whether we think that it has areas where nurses can act as independent practitioners. In addition other factors have been shown to be of importance in assessing, planning and giving care, such as the age of the patient, whether he is likely to be in hospital for a short or long time, and whether his admission was planned or an emergency. Only evaluation stayed the same throughout.

Now let us examine yet another variable which will affect the assessment, planning and giving of nursing care, and that is the setting in which the patient is being nursed. The greater part of nurse training still takes place in hospital, but all nurses will soon be expected to have at least some experience of what the EEC directives call 'home nursing', though it is more familiar to us as 'community nursing' or in its postbasic form as district nursing and health visiting. It is the use of the nursing process in community nursing which we are now going to examine, looking first at the way in which district nurses may be observed to be using it and then at the way in which it will influence the work of the health visitor.

District Nursing

The use of the nursing process by district nurses is as much influenced by their approach to nursing as this approach influences the kind of care given by nurses working in any other setting. In other words, some district nurses see themselves very much as doctors' assistants, while others value their independent function more. However, the current district nursing curriculum comes down firmly on the side of the district nurse as an independent practitioner, though cooperating closely with members of the primary health care team and with other health and welfare workers. Nurse learners in the future should therefore be able to discern this trend in the way in which district nurses assess patient needs, as well as in the way in which they plan and give care. Nevertheless, the basic phases of the process remain immutable, and it is to these that we shall now address ourselves.

Assessment

Assessment, as we remember, includes collecting as much useful information about the patient as possible as a basis for planning care. The information comes from records, observation and interviews. District nurses get their information by similar means, though their sources will differ.

Records

Let us first of all look at records. People are usually entered on the list of a general practitioner soon after birth, unless they are born abroad or belong to that small percentage of the population who still consult a doctor privately. Persons born before the inception of the National Health Service were registered with general practitioners after 1948. For every person so registered the local Family Practitioner Committee provides the general practitioner with a record card and an envelope in which to keep it together with any other pertinent information about the patient (the status usually occupied by persons who go to see their doctor). Should a person move away from the area in which his doctor lives or should he wish to change doctor for any other reason, his records are returned to the Family Practitioner Committee and reissued by it to the new doctor with whom the patient indicates his wish to register. This means that for the majority of patients whom district nurses are asked to visit extensive records exist within general practice. Attachment schemes have made these records available to district nurses, and they are usually consulted before a nurse first visits a new patient. If relevant, district nurses may also consult records of other members of the patient's family or household for information. In a growing number of cases records do not confine themselves any more only to doctors' notes, but other members of the primary health care team may either use the same record sheet or keep their separate record cards in the same place as medical records.

Therefore the records available to district nurses differ considerably from those which nurses in hospital usually refer to. They should provide a health and treatment biography of the patient, though in practice primary health care team members may be as fallible about record-keeping as anyone else. On the other hand, they may lack records of recent detailed scientific investigations often contained in patients' notes in hospital, for access to laboratory facilities is restricted in many instances.

Because of the length of time many patients have been on their general practitioner's list it is quite possible that they may be known not only to the doctor but to the receptionist or, perhaps, to the health visitor. In many instances the learner may be able to observe the district nurse making enquiries about her new patient from these people so that she may go on her first visit with as much background information as possible. Such information is not collected from a sense of inquisitiveness, but because it may prove genuinely helpful later on when care has to be planned.

Observation

Armed with much useful information, the district nurse will now use the more direct forms of data gathering available to her, namely observation and interview. In practice, it is difficult to disentangle these two, for many observations will be made during the course of interviewing, and many questions become unnecessary if the nurse uses her eyes carefully.

However, in district nursing observations will have to be made not only with regard to the patient, but in relation to the environment in which he is found. While – as we saw especially in the chapter on care-giving – the structure and equipment of the ward do affect nursing care, once they have been assessed they stay the same for all patients. This is contrary to what happens in district nursing, where not only the patient but his environment will have to be observed anew every time. As we already know, in detail, about observations as they affect the patient, let us concentrate on observations made with regard to the environment: first, with the immediate environment of the patient and, from there, to the wider environment in which the patient resides, and which may also affect his nursing care.

It may be appropriate to begin by observing the patient's clothing, whether he be in bed or up and about. The quantity as well as the quality of clothing can tell us something about the patient, his heat regulating mechanism, his economic circumstances, or the cultural influences which helped in shaping his personality. There are also more covert cues: a person sitting by a fire wearing a dressing gown and slippers may indicate that he has no intention to venture out of doors, while another with a cardigan stained and fastened incorrectly may signal anything from shortsightedness to mental confusion. Of course, these are only indicators or cues, and cannot stand as diagnostic inferences without further corroborating evidence, but they should not be ignored.

Furniture and furnishings can tell their own story but should not be taken merely as evidence of financial status, taste or cleanliness. They may well have an important part to play as therapeutic instruments. For some reason, not so far investigated, many sick persons are moved from their usual sleeping accommodation, often to a living room and frequently into a single bed. Domestic bedsteads are usually of a height which facilitates sitting on the edge and getting up, but they may be uncomfortably low for nursing a patient for any length of time. On the whole though, the question of height assumes far greater importance when applied to chairs, for many easy chairs are just that, easy to sit in but almost impossible to get out of without considerable physical effort, and thus may present problems for people who are in any way handicapped, and who sometimes are unnecessarily restrained through them in their independence. Equally important, however, are observations related to the amount of furniture in a room, and the position of the bed. It is difficult for a righthanded person to assist a patient from the left side of the bed. It is equally difficult for a person with, for example, right-sided hemiplegia, to have to get out of bed on the right side of the bed or to have to have his drink, paper handkerchiefs and spectacles placed on that side. Floor covering, whether carpet, mats, highly polished lino or wood all bring their own problems. Unlike the hospital, few beds can be approached from both sides. Generally speaking, overcrowded rooms are going to present difficulties as much for the patient as for the carers.

Observations should also be directed towards the arrangement of the house or flat in general. What about the situation of washing and toilet facilities? Are there any possible causes for accidents such as loose mats? The learner may well notice that the district nurse does not necessarily ask direct questions about these things, but makes her observations while washing her hands or collecting some piece of equipment. Nor will it always be necessary to find the answers to all these questions at the first visit, particularly where it is anticipated that care will have to be given for some time. But these answers *should* be found at some time; moreover, such answers *should* be recorded.

Observations of the wider environment, which will be included in any nursing assessment made by district nurses, are things like the approach to the house or flat – Are there stairs to negotiate and, if so, are there handrails in situ? Is there a garden and, if so, is it well kept or neglected? Does it provide facilities for drying the washing? What about shops? Are they close by, and are they easily accessible, or are they, perhaps, on the other side of a busy main road? What about a launderette or a pub or a park?

Let us at this point move from the account of some of the information which will be available through observation and which will have to be collected on any new patient being nursed in his own home. However, we must bear in mind that not all this information may have to be collected at one visit, nor will it all necessarily have to be collected from every patient, nor may it all have to be acted upon for every patient. But much of it is useful, and most of it is easily available.

Interviewing

Interviewing, or asking questions of the patient, has the same purpose at home as anywhere else. It helps to establish a base line, to find out the patient's present knowledge, his attitude to his condition, and his aspirations for the future. It also tells us such things of his past as will account for his present unique disposition. However, looking at the questions which have to be asked at home, it may well become apparent that they may be fewer, for much of the information that has to be collected about a person's lifestyle by interview when he is away from his normal environment will be self-evident in his home, and can there be collected by observation.

Patients in hospital, as many of us know, often give somewhat inaccurate information about how they will manage at home and the help that will be available to them there. Part of the assessment process at home will consist of observing and interviewing not only the patient but those who will be responsible for his care during the time that the district nurse will not be present. That person's physical, mental and intellectual state will also have to be assessed. A decision will often have to be taken whether assessing those responsible for patient care in the absence of the nurse should take place at the same time and in the presence of the patient or separately.

When as much information as possible has been collected by consultation of records, observations and interviews, problem identification can begin. However, while the majority of problems identified in hospital will belong to the patient, in the community nursing problems may be patient problems, or they may equally well reside in the physical environment, in the social and economic conditions of the patient or, most importantly, in the carer who may be unable or unwilling to take up the responsibility of the carer role. We know that problems may be actual or potential; they may, however, in community care be problems of the home environment as much as of patient and may be family rather than individual ones. As previously indicated, problems which have been identified should be checked with patient and carers, that is, they should be validated.

Planning Patient Care

Having identified as many problems as possible, plans for meeting them will have to be made. There will be a hierarchy of needs, from planning for potentially life-threatening situations to problems which, while enriching the patients' or their carers' lifestyle, may be seen as luxuries for which no resources can be spared. The plans which are made will again depend on what we consider nursing to be, but, in district nursing particularly, plans will have to differentiate between ideal and possible plans. District nurses will often be found to formulate ideal plans first; however, after checking them against not only the resources which are available within their own service but also those which can be mustered by the patient they will have to be modified.

Problems may have to be divided into those which are not amenable to any intervention, those which are amenable to intervention by the patient and lay carers, those which are amenable to nursing intervention, those where other members of the primary health care team may have to be involved, and those which will necessitate the involvement of other agencies. From the nursing point of view the district nurse will have to decide who will be the most appropriate member of her team to tackle a particular problem. She will have to state her goals in such a way that they are observable and thus appropriate for evaluation.

The setting of goals is as difficult in district nursing as in any other situation, not only because it is sometimes difficult to set the goals so that they can be observed but because knowing what goals are appropriate will require a thorough knowledge of human physiology and pathology, as well as an appreciation of social and emotional factors which may motivate people in achieving their maximum potential. The making of goals too hard to achieve may bring despondency to patient, carer and nurse, but making them too easy may mean that the patient is not getting the best out of life. Sometimes district nurses have to learn to live with the frustrations of knowing that the patient could do better if only he wanted to, and more frequently that he could do more for himself if only his carers were not being overprotective.

It will be absolutely vital for the district nurse to agree on the goals that are to be achieved and their means of achievement with the patient and his carers, for unlike hospital staff, carers at home are not under the control of nurses and do not *have* to do as they are told. However, the majority are only too anxious to do anything in their power to help provided they fully understand what is expected of them.

Not only will the district nurse have to teach and guide and support the patient and his lay carers, but she will have to do the same with her nursing team. She will have to make sure that, should she decide to delegate some part of a patient's care, the goals agreed upon between herself and the patient and carers are clearly understood and respected, as well as the way in which they are to be achieved. Furthermore, she must agree contingencies which would necessitate referral back to her for amendment of plans.

Implementation of Care Plans

In many instances nursing is seen as doing things for or with a patient, but in district nursing there is a much greater emphasis on seeing that things get done than on the nurse doing them herself. After all, there are very few instances where the nurse will be with a patient for as much as even two hours a day, and in many instances she may only see him weekly or even monthly. However, whatever the frequency of her visit, she is ultimately responsible for the nursing care given to the patient. She may therefore have only a relatively small 'nursing' input in the way that nursing is often understood, that is in carrying out actual treatments. But she will have a much larger input particularly of teaching and of checking that her teaching has been understood and has also been carried out. Because many patients who are not nursed in hospital may have long-term illnesses, these may be very trying to the patient as well as to all those who care for him. The nurse's role in these situations may well be that of giving support to the patient and his family, assuring them that they are doing well and that professional care could not achieve results superior to their own. They may also often have to help everyone to come to terms with chronic disability or impending death. In these instances the district nurse may act as guide to sources of help and relief, financial as well as personal. It may be that, while the patient himself is doing well, the family situation around him is breaking up, and support may have to be given to those not ostensibly patients at all. All in all, nurse learners may often be surprised by the large amount of talking there is in community nursing care compared with the relatively small amount of technical care, but whatever actions she observes these should find their rationale in the nursing care plan, or else the plan should be amended to take account of a changing situation.

Evaluation

Evaluation is particularly important in community nursing, and especially in district nursing, where many patients have chronic or long-term illnesses. Without evaluation, which should take place at regular intervals and not only when a patient is discharged or dies, it is quite possible for changes to occur so gradually that they may be missed. Sometimes the changes are in the patient or the carer, but at others they may be in the care which is being given, and which has been adjusted to meet changing needs without anyone consciously noticing it. If no note has been made of such changes in the care plan, relief and holiday nurses may not be aware of them, and the patient may either have to instruct the nurse himself (with the nurse feeling unsure of whether or not she is doing the right thing) or he may receive inappropriate care.

The use of the nursing process in district nursing indicates the similarities between nursing in hospital and in patients' own homes and also shows up the very real differences that exist between these two forms of nursing. By being alert, particularly to the latter, it is hoped that nurse learners will derive maximum benefit from their community experience.

Health Visiting

Nurse learners often have difficulty in understanding the work of health visitors; a brief introduction to that work is essential before showing the way in which nursing process can be applied to it. Health visitors are nurses primarily concerned with the promotion and maintainance of health and the prevention of ill health;

they provide this service to individuals and families in the community.

The health visitors differ from the hospital and district nurses in that they work predominantly with well people. Hospital and district nurses usually refer to the recipients of care as *patients* whereas health visitors use the term *client* because patient is too reminiscent of being sick. This change in terminology may seem a little strange when visiting families with the health visitor for the first time.

Whom Does the Health Visitor Visit?

The health visitor, as we now know, works with well individuals and families in the community. Ideally the health visitor would like to visit every person or family in her area or registered with the general practitioner with whom she works at regular intervals, since everybody is at risk of developing certain health problems which may be identified and perhaps ameliorated or prevented by regular visiting. However, in some individuals the risk of developing problems is increased. A person's potential for health is determined, broadly speaking, by three factors:

1. Genetic makeup
2. Lifestyle
3. Environmental factors

Genetic makeup

Each individual has his or her own unique genetic makeup which to a limited extent determines the individual's potential for growth and development. The health visitor cannot change the genetic endowment of a person but may be able to help a family or individual plan to attain the maximum potential for healthy living within the constraints of their genetic makeup. For example,

> A child may be born deaf; however, early detection of the deafness by the health visitor may enable the child and parents to receive help and guidance from experts.

Lifestyle

The style of life one leads has an important impact on health. Poor dietary habits, such as eating a predominantly carbohydrate diet, are known to cause obesity, which may predispose to heart disease, varicose veins and other conditions of varying severity. Again the health visitor cannot change a person's eating habits, for the client is ultimately responsible for his own life. The health visitor, however, may be instrumental in helping the client to recognise the potential problem inherent in eating a poor diet. Recognition of the problem may stimulate the client to modify his own behaviour, in this case his eating habits.

Environmental factors
The environment in which a person lives influences health and well-being. The environment may be considered in two ways: first, the individual environment or home and, second, the wider environment or community.

We know from history that living in overcrowded poorly ventilated conditions encourages the transmission of infectious diseases, especially airborne infections such as tuberculosis, diphtheria and even the common cold. The health visitor used to be very much involved in the management of infectious diseases. Today, legislation has altered the picture by setting minimum standards regarding ventilation and overcrowding, hence the modern health visitor is more involved in primary prevention, such as immunization, rather than advising on the management and prevention of spread of the established disease. The wider environment or community also exerts its influence on the health of individuals. Again history has shown that clean water supplies and adequate sanitation improve the health of individuals and hence the community.

What Does the Health Visitor Do?
Health visitors have a responsibility to provide a service to families with children under five years of age. Since health visitors have been attached to general practice they have had more contact with other age groups such as the elderly and middle aged. General practice attachment provides the health visitor with a readily accessible pool of people from which she may select those most at risk of developing health problems. The search for persons with actual and potential health problems is a unique feature of health visiting.

To the nurse learner it may appear that the health visitor does very little apart from looking at babies, and talking. Doing in nursing is sometimes linked with performing tasks. In the section on district nursing we note that the learner may think that the district nurse does more talking than the hospital nurse; the health visitor probably does even more talking in relation to doing than the district nurse. To the uninitiated the work of the health visitor could be interpreted as 'just talking to people'. However, it is the content of the conversation which is important. The content of the health visitor's conversation may differ from that of the district nurse and hospital nurse; by placing emphasis on the content of the conversation the learner may find the key to understanding the health visitor's work.

The health visitor, unlike the district nurse, does not usually visit clients by arrangement; some visits may be carried out at the request of the client but most are not. The reason for this is that the health visitor is involved in searching out potential as well as actual health problems. Although the district nurse and hospital nurse may identify potential health problems and act upon them their first contact with the patient is usually brought about because the patient has an actual health problem. Some of the clients the health visitor visits may have no actual problems though many potential problems. Many clients do not share the health visitors' knowledge of health and its related factors, so that health visitors devote a good deal of their time to health education, which involves sharing information and knowledge with clients in the hope that they will become more aware of the factors related to the achievement of optimum health.

Prevention

Prevention may be subdivided into three phases: primary, secondary and tertiary. The health visitor may become involved at any of these levels with a client. In order to explain the three kinds of prevention an illustration may help taking one health problem through all three stages. The problem:

> Smoking is said to predispose towards chest infections and lung cancer, as well as to other conditions of varying severity.

Primary prevention   The aim of primary prevention in this example is to reduce the number of persons who smoke; to prevent non-smokers becoming smokers and to change existing smokers into non-smokers. Unfortunately, there is no easily available solution to the problem. If we wished to eradicate poliomyelitis we could immunise large numbers of people and eventually the organism causing the disease would become extinct. Because there is no proven way to reduce the numbers of people who smoke the current approach is health education.

The aim of antismoking programmes is to provide people with the information they need so that they can make informed decision about smoking; some people may never smoke and others who already smoke may give it up. This then reduces the number of people at risk from developing lung cancer through smoking and is one way of attempting to prevent the disease.

Secondary prevention   Secondary prevention is concerned with the early detection of disease. To continue with the example on smoking, the health visitor may be concerned about a client's cough and advise the client to go to the doctor. The doctor may examine the patient and diagnose bronchitis and prescribe the necessary treatment, advise the client to give up smoking. If the client had not been prompted to seek early medical attention the bronchitis might have become more severe and resulted in an extreme case in chronic lung damage.

Tertiary prevention   Tertiary prevention is the area in which the health visitor is least involved, and can also be termed *rehabilitation*. The disease process has run its full course and the health visitor attempts to assist the individual to maintain or acquire his maximum level of health and well-being. The end result for some smokers is lung cancer, sometimes resulting in extensive chest surgery. In tertiary prevention the health visitor might become involved with her client after he has recovered physically from surgery; she could perhaps assist the client and his family to come to terms with the social and psychological effects of cancer.

Using the problem of smoking and lung cancer we have tried to give the learner an understanding of the three levels of prevention, though it is acknowledged that factors other than smoking may determine if an individual will contract lung cancer.

So far we have identified that health visitors are nurses working predominantly with well people; they have a responsibility to families with children under five years of age, although they do visit other age groups. The health visitors are involved in three levels of prevention and search out and identify clients with actual and potential health problems; they deal with their clients' problems by using their skills as health educators; these skills often manifest themselves in the content of the health visitor's conversation.

How Health Visitors Use the Nursing Process

The health visitors in carrying out their duties can use all the stages of the nursing process covered in the preceding chapters.

Assessment

Assessment is similar to that used by other nurses in that it involves the collection of information; however, the information collected may be different from that collected by the district and hospital nurse. Health visitors draw upon their knowledge of normal development throughout the life cycle and on their knowledge of the physical, social, psychological and environmental factors known to predispose towards health problems. It is from this perspective that the health visitor begins to collect information from her client or with her client. The factors which contribute towards mental, physical and social well-being, we know, are: genetic makeup, lifestyle and environment. The health visitor conducts her assessment in the clinic or in the home as does the district nurse, and an assessment is not considered to be complete unless the client's home has been visited.

The health visitor is also involved in another type of assessment which is referred to as 'community assessment'. The health visitor needs to know the resources available in the community, the common problems of the community and the future needs of the community. The means which the health visitor employs to collect her data are the same as those used by other nurses, namely: search of records, consultation, interviewing and observation. Some of the information the health visitor extracts from records may be similar to that extracted by other nurses; but the information which she obtains through other means such as interview will probably differ because it may be related to preventive health measures and not illness related matters.

The district nurse and health visitor will both assess the furniture in a person's home. The district nurse may view a chair for its potential therapeutic use: 'Is this chair too high or too low for my patient to sit on?'

The health visitor primarily assesses the furniture and its location from a safety perspective; a chair under an open window may present a health hazard in a home with a child.

This does not mean that the health visitor might not assess the therapeutic use of a chair and the district nurse its safety aspects, but the emphasis may well be different.

Validation

Validating a problem with a client is of particular importance in health visiting, because it is usually the client who deals with the problem and not the health visitor. If a client does *not* acknowledge a potential or actual problem then it is difficult and sometimes impossible to deal with it.

Planning care

Planning care is relatively easy when dealing with individuals. However, the health visitor is usually involved with families which means identifying the actual and potential health problems of each family member and determining where possible their interrelationship. Goals have to be set for the solution of each health problem and appropriate plans made. Some problems may be more important or immediate than others and a hierarchy may be established to enable the more important problems to be dealt with first.

An infant feeding problem is potentially life-threatening and should be dealt with before a problem related to development.

In the case of interrelated problems a nursing action may solve more than one problem:

A mother may tell the health visitor that her baby is always hungry and cries continually after feeds. The health visitor may observe the baby feeding on several occasions and not hear the baby cry, but notices that the mother appears very tense. This may lead her to suspect that the feeding problem is a symptom of another problem. On further discussion with the mother it may transpire that she is having difficulties in her sex life because she is frightened of becoming pregnant again.

In this example, advice on family planning and if necessary a referral to the family planning clinic may solve both problems.

The learners, who probably have had more experience in planning care for the sick who may be unable to act for themselves, should bear in mind that planning care for the well *is* different. It is usually the client or family who decides if the care plan is appropriate and who usually puts it into practice, therefore it is of paramount importance to include the client in planning at every stage.

If a client has a potential problem of an unwanted pregnancy, the health visitor may give advice about contraception. However, inevitably the client decides what line of action to take; whether the male or female partner will take responsibility for contraception, whether to attend a family planning clinic or the general practitioner.

The health visitor provides the information which the client will need in order to make an informed decision.

The client or family should when possible be involved in goal-setting, since, once again, it is the client who is often the first to know if the goal has been achieved.

Goal statement: The child will use the potty or toilet each time he urinates or has his bowels opened.

Plan: Reward the child with praise and a cuddle each time he uses the potty or toilet, and then withhold praise if he fails to use the potty or toilet.

In this example it will probably be the child's parents who will be the first to know when the child has reached the goal and become fully continent. The health visitor usually relies upon the parents for feedback since she has no other reliable way of obtaining the information.

Sharing is an important concept in nursing. The health visitor shares information with the client and discusses her perception of the client's problem with him. There is a mutual exchange of information, but the client always retains the ultimate responsibility for his own health. It may be helpful to view the health visitor as an enabler who provides information to help the client or family plan to attain their own optimum level of health and well-being.

Evaluation

Evaluation is fundamentally the same in health visiting as it is in other areas of nursing. Criteria are established usually of a behavioural nature and evaluation dates set; a comparison is made between the expected outcome and the achieved outcome. In hospital the patient may be clearly defined as the person receiving nursing care and the goals are usually specific to the patient. However in community nursing and in particular in health visiting the effect of health visitor intervention may have to be evaluated not only for individuals but also for families. The health visitor may have to work at any one time with large numbers of goals some of which may be conflicting. Because the health visitor has relatively infrequent contact with her clients compared to the hospital and district nurse she has to rely quite heavily on the client to evaluate for her.

Through this brief introduction to health visiting and the nursing process, we hope to make the nurse learners' community experience, in particular, their time spent with the health visitor, more meaningful, and to focus their concentration on the content of the health visitor's conversation and make their own comparisons with other types of nursing.

164

Suggested Reading

Barefoot P. & P. J. Cunningham (1977) *Community Services: The Health Worker's A to Z.* London: Faber & Faber.

CETHV (1977) *An Investigation into the Principles of Health Visiting.* London: CETHV.

Clark J. (1973) *A Family Visitor. A Descriptive Analysis of Health Visiting in Berkshire.* London: Royal College of Nursing.

Hicks D. (1976) *Primary Health Care.* London: HMSO.

McIntosh, J. B. (1979) The nurse-patient relationship. *Nursing Mirror Supplement*, January 25, pp. i-xi.

Owen G. M. (1977) *Health Visiting.* London: Baillière Tindall.

Index

Index

167